Comorbidity in Migraine

Comorbidity in Migraine

EDITED BY

Jean Schoenen MD PhD
Professor of Functional Neuroanatomy
and Clinical Professor of Neurology
Department of Neurology & GIGA-Neurosciences
Liège University
Liège, Belgium

David W. Dodick MD
Professor of Neurology
Department of Neurology
Mayo Clinic Arizona
Phoenix, AZ, USA

Peter S. Sándor MD
Chief of Neurology
Cantonal Hospital of Baden
RehaClinic Zurzach
University of Zürich
Baden Dätwill, Switzerland

WILEY-BLACKWELL

A John Wiley & Sons, Ltd., Publication

Library of Congress Cataloging-in-Publication Data

Comorbidity in migraine/edited by Jean Schoenen, David W. Dodick, Peter S. Sandor.
    p. ; cm.
  Includes bibliographical references and index.
  ISBN 978-1-4051-8555-4 (alk. paper)
1. Migraine. 2. Comorbidity. I. Schoenan, Jean. II. Dodick, David. III. Sandor, Peter S.
  [DNLM: 1. Migraine Disorders–epidemiology. 2. Comorbidity. WL 344]
  RC392.C656 2011
  616.8′4912–dc22

                                            2010038308

ISBN: 978-1-4051-8555-4

This is book is published in the following electronic formats: ePDF 9781444328387; Wiley Online Library 9781444328370

A catalogue record for this book is available from the British Library.

Set in 9.25/11.5pt Minion by SPi Publisher Services, Pondicherry, India
Printed and bound in Singapore by Fabulous Printers Pte Ltd

2 2012

Contents

Preface, vi

List of Contributors, viii

1 Psychiatric Comorbidity in Migraine, 1
Françoise Radat, Amanda Kalaydjian and Kathleen R. Merikangas

2 Migraine and Stroke, 14
Tobias Kurth and Hans-Christoph Diener

3 Cardiovascular Disorders, 27
Ann I. Scher and David W. Dodick

4 Patent Foramen Ovale and Migraine, 41
Todd J. Schwedt and Jean Schoenen

5 Comorbidity of Migraine and Epilepsy, 59
Sheryl Haut, Shira Markowitz and Richard B. Lipton

6 Migraine and Other Pain Disorders, 81
Lars Jacob Stovner, Knut Hagen and Rami Burstein

7 Migraine and Medication Overuse, 96
Stephen D. Silberstein

8 Migraine and Other Comorbidities: Obesity, Temporomandibular Disorders and Contact Points, 112
Marcelo E. Bigal

9 Migraine Comorbidities in Children, 122
Çiçek Wöber-Bingöl and Andrew Hershey

10 Optimal Management of Migraine Taking Into Account Comorbidities and 'Positive Side Effects', 132
Peter S. Sándor, David W. Dodick and Jean Schoenen

Index, 138

Preface

Comorbidity is defined as a condition that occurs more frequently in association with a specific disorder than would be found as a coincidental association in the general population. There at least three reasons why comorbidity is of interest in migraine and why a book on the present state of knowledge can be valuable.

First, migraine, partly because of its high prevalence, is likely to be among the disorders with the highest rate of comorbidity. Besides the well documented and consistent association with psychiatric disorders, stroke and epilepsy in population-based studies, recent findings suggest that up to 21 somatic conditions may be comorbid with migraine, especially in women and migraine with aura. Among them, allergies, thrombosis, low back and neck pain, fibromyalgia, osteoporosis, lupus, psoriatic and rheumatoid arthritis, thyroid disease and Menière's disease.

Second, identifying and understanding the basis for comorbidity between migraine and another disorder may shed light on the etiopathogenesis of migraine and pave the way for novel research paths or therapeutic approaches. Comorbidity with stroke draws attention to potential vascular factors in migraine pathophysiology, comorbidity with immunopathological disorders to possible auto-immune mechanisms, comorbid pain disorders to the role of pain control systems and comorbidity with psychiatric disease and epilepsy to that of cortical and subcortical networks and neurotransmitter dysfunction. The causal relationship between migraine and a comorbid disorder may be multiple and complex, ranging from shared genetic components to common environmental factors. In most instances, the basis for these relationships is not well understood and clearly needs further research.

Last, but not least, migraine comorbidities also have immediate and practical aspects. The prognosis and management of migraine is strongly influenced by the presence of comorbid disorders and the risk of developing such disorders. The choice of an anti-migraine treatment must take into account comorbidities and vice versa. Especially for the preventive treatment, a good selection of substances has the potential to treat simultaneously migraine and the comorbid disorder, which can improve patient compliance considerably.

For all these reasons, we found it timely to collect comprehensive reviews from a number of distinguished experts in the field to whom we are deeply indebted. The resulting book offers a synoptic review of the most important disorders which may be comorbid with migraine. Illustrative clinical presentations are added for each of them, as "problem-solving" case reports.

The prevalence and risk ratios for comorbid disorders are presented on the basis of available epidemiologic data. Pathophysiological links and susceptibility models to explain the comorbid relationship are critically analyzed. Finally, management strategies are proposed for migraine in the presence of each comorbid disorder, and, in the final chapter, we present a model strategy for the optimal management both of migraine and the comorbid disorder taking into account available preventive migraine treatments and their side effect profiles.

This book is intended for the broad array of clinicians involved in the care of patients with headache including headache experts, neurologists, primary care physicians, psychiatrists, and others. Most importantly, we hope that this book will inform your clinical-decision making and be of value to you and your patients, and … that it will also be fun reading it.

Jean Schoenen, David Dodick & Peter Sándor
Liège, Phoenix and Zurich

List of Contributors

Marcelo E. Bigal

Merck Research Laboratories, Whitehouse Station, NJ, USA; and Department of Neurology, Albert Einstein College of Medicine, NY, USA

Rami Burstein

Department of Anesthesia and Critical Care, Beth Israel Deaconess Medical Center, Harvard Medical School, Boston, MA, USA

Hans-Christophe Diener

Department of Neurology, University of Duisburg-Essen, Essen, Germany

Knut Hagen

Norwegian National Headache Centre, Department of Neuroscience, Norwegian University of Science and Technology and St Olav's Hospital, Trondheim, Norway

Sheryl Haut

Adult Epilepsy Service, Montefiore Medical Center, Albert Einstein College of Medicine, NY, USA

Andrew Hershey

Department of Pediatrics, Division of Neurology, Cincinnati Children's Hospital Medical Center and University of Cincinnati College of Medicine, Cincinnati, OH, USA; Jefferson Headache Center, Thomas Jefferson University Hospital, Philadelphia, PA, USA

Amanda Kalaydjian

Intramural Research Program, National Institute of Mental Health, Falls Church, VA, USA

Tobias Kurth

Faculty of Medicine, University Pierre et Marie Curie, Paris, France; Division of Preventive Medicine, Brigham and Women's Hospital, Harvard Medical School and Department of Epidemiology, Harvard School of Public Health, Boston, MA, USA

Richard B. Lipton

Department of Epidemiology and Population Health, Albert Einstein College of Medicine and Montefiore Headache Unit, NY, USA

Shira Markowitz

Department of Neurology, Albert Einstein College of Medicine, NY, USA

Kathleen R. Merikangas

Intramural Research Program, National Institute of Mental Health, Falls Church, VA, USA

Françoise Radat
Chronic Pain Treatment Unit, University Hospital, Bordeaux, France

Ann I. Scher
Department of Preventive Medicine and Biometrics, Uniformed Services University, Bethesda, MD, USA

Todd J. Schwedt
Washington University Headache Center, Washington University School of Medicine, St Louis, MO, USA

Stephen D. Silberstein
Jefferson Headache Center, Thomas Jefferson University Hospital, Philadelphia, PA, USA

Lars J. Stovner
Norwegian National Headache Centre, Department of Neuroscience, Norwegian University of Science and Technology and St. Olavs Hospital, Trondheim, Norway

Çiçek Wöber-Bingöl
Department of Psychiatry of Childhood and Adolescence, Medical University of Vienna, Vienna, Austria

1 Psychiatric Comorbidity in Migraine

Françoise Radat[1], Amanda Kalaydjian[2] & Kathleen R. Merikangas[2]
[1] Chronic Pain Treatment Unit, University Hospital, Bordeaux, France
[2] Intramural Research Program, National Institute of Mental Health, Falls Church, VA, USA

Introduction

The association of migraine with various psychological characteristics such as depressive tendencies, perfectionism and autonomic reactivity has been described by clinicians for more than a century. There is now abundant evidence from numerous large, population-based studies across a wide range of geographic sites that people with migraine have greater rates of mood and anxiety disorders. The data generated from such studies have also demonstrated the impact of comorbidity on the onset, course and severity of migraine, as well as use of services and response to treatment.

The goals of this chapter are to review: (i) the epidemiological evidence of psychiatric comorbidity in migraine; (ii) empirical evidence regarding the possible underlying mechanisms of these associations; (iii) the effects of psychiatric comorbidity on migraine course, severity and response to treatment; and (iv) the consideration of comorbidity in determining treatment for migraine patients. A case report illustrates the complex issues of psychiatric comorbidity.

Case report

Miss E. is 24 years old. She has been suffering from migraine without aura since adolescence. She consults now because her illness has become very incapacitating; for more than 6 months she has been experiencing one or more migraine attacks per week that persisted for two or three days. On those days, she takes one or two tablets of a combination anti-inflammatory and barbiturate, but she has begun taking these tablets more often during the past year. Therefore, medication overuse headache (MOH) is suspected. Her anxiety during the interview is impressive, and she confirms that she is currently 'stressed'. She is preparing for a competitive examination and has had difficulty concentrating on her work because of her headaches. She does not sleep well, ruminating during the night over what she could not do during the day. She suffers from guilt and accuses herself of having a 'lack of willpower'.

Comorbidity in Migraine, First Edition. Edited by J. Schoenen, D. W. Dodick and P. S. Sándor.
© 2011 Blackwell Publishing Ltd. Published 2011 by Blackwell Publishing Ltd.

Miss E. describes a history of anxiety since childhood. Her anxiety is generally focused on usual life stresses but she becomes far more anxious than she feels is warranted by the focal situation. Aside from anxiety, she has had excellent social and educational functioning. She reports brief, mild depressive episodes beginning at about age 16, with a first episode of depression occurring at the break-up of a relationship at age 18. She also reports periods of feeling better than usual during which she has more energy, is more active and sleeps two to three hours less per night. These periods last about four to five days and she returns to her usual pattern of sleep and activity afterwards. Her family history includes an alcoholic maternal grandfather and a mother's puerperal depression following birth of the patient's younger sister.

Miss E.'s headaches seem to have progressively worsened over the last three years. During this time, she has suffered from hypersomnia, abulia and anhedonia that persisted for about six months. Miss E. was treated with amitriptyline (75 mg/day) during the previous year but she became agitated and had a weight gain of about 12 kg over the past six months. Currently, she is being treated with atenolol (80 mg/day), but has not been taking the treatment for more than a month because it made her 'sleep too much'.

Overall, this young patient presents with migraine without aura, exacerbated by the onset of possible medication overuse headache during the past six months. The disorder worsened since she began to have depression, which was determined to be of moderate severity. On account of the family history of alcoholism and current medication overuse, there is a need for assessment of dependence on acute antimigraine drugs and other substances. The possible history of hypomanic episodes, anxiety disorders, and major depressive episodes, when considered together with her family history of maternal puerperal major depression and alcoholism in the paternal grandfather, raise concerns about bipolar mood disorder.

Association of migraine with affective disorders

Clinical and population studies of migraine have documented a two- to four-fold increase in mood disorders in people with migraine compared to those without migraine Table 1.1 [1–16]. Rates of comorbidity are far greater in clinical settings than in the general population. Studies of patients in tertiary care centres indicate that approximately 50% exhibit a significant increase in current depression scores [17,18]. Migraine may also predispose to more severe depression as the risk of suicide is greater in migraine than non-migraine patients even after controlling for the existence of depression [1,19]. The association between migraine and the bipolar subtype of depression has been reported to be greater than that for major depressive disorder alone; however, the lower prevalence of the bipolar subtype in many studies diminishes the power to discriminate differences across mood disorder subtypes [1,6,9,15,16,20–22]. Regardless, given the substantial comorbidity of migraine with mood disorders, it is imperative for clinicians to evaluate migraine patients for the presence of depressive and manic symptoms in order to design a treatment regimen that can treat both disorders if necessary.

Migraine patients do not always spontaneously express their depressive complaints, which they readily ascribe to their headaches if they are frequent. As a matter of fact, depressive cognitions are often related to pain ('I am totally unreliable because of my migraine'; 'Things will never be better'…). If the patients are reluctant to accept the diagnostic of depression, the physician can rely on symptoms such as sleep disorders, lack of energy and loss of interest to have the patients accept the diagnostic.

Association of migraine with anxiety disorders

Anxiety disorders may have an even stronger association with migraine than mood disorders. There is a two- to six-fold increased risk for aggregate anxiety disorders as well as subtypes thereof among migraine sufferers compared with those without migraine Table 1.1. With respect to specific subtypes of anxiety disorders, panic attacks and disorder appear to have the strongest association with migraine, followed by phobic disorders and generalized anxiety disorder [1,2,5–7,9,11,12,15,16,23]. Perfectionism and obsessionality have been reported in clinical descriptions of people with migraine, but few studies have systematically evaluated this association. Although Breslau et al. [1] found that the prevalence of obsessive compulsive disorder was associated with migraine in the general population, this association has not been confirmed in several other studies [5,9]. The well-established co-occurrence of anxiety and depression has also been observed in population studies of people with migraine [10,24]. In general, the onset of anxiety in people with migraine is reported to occur in childhood and adolescence, but there is no evidence that anxiety occurs earlier among those with migraine in population surveys.

Anxiety in migraine patients mainly focuses on the fear of a new attack, which can induce the development of exaggerated avoiding behaviours towards trigger factors in phobic patients. Stress, by the way, is considered as a classical trigger factor for migraine attacks. Anticipating anxiety can also be a factor facilitating the development of medication overuse, when the patient takes medication at the slightest sign of a possible impending attack. Finally, some patients may develop panic attacks at the time of occurrence of migraine attacks if migraine headaches had previously been symptomatic of a serious event such as, for instance, a meningeal hemorrhage.

Association of migraine with substance dependence

The association between migraine and substance use disorders is somewhat contradictory. The increased odds of dependence on nicotine, alcohol and illicit drugs in subjects with migraine reported by Breslau et al. [1] was not replicated in most other studies [9,15,16] Table 1.1. Some of the discrepant findings may be attributable to the lack of discrimination between licit and illicit drugs. People with migraine are at increased risk to develop abuse of drugs used to treat migraine such as painkillers and barbiturates. Around two-thirds of patients suffering from medication overuse headache are dependent on acute antimigraine drugs according to the DSM-IV (Diagnostic and Statistical Manual of Mental Disorders IV) diagnostic criteria for behavioural loss of control of drug consumption and compulsive intake [25,26]. Migraine patients' susceptibility to addiction, and even that of their relatives, as suggested by the existence of dependence on licit substances (tobacco, anxiolytics, alcohol), might be a risk factor for the development of MOH [27]. The majority of studies show, however, that there is no association between alcohol use disorders and migraine.

Migraine and personality traits

Although the clinical literature provides numerous descriptions of the personality of patients with migraine, there has been limited empirical evidence for an association between migraine and either personality disorders or a specific constellation of personality traits [28]. Those studies that do purport to link personality traits to migraine suffer from several methodological shortcomings including: the lack of representative samples; absence of a control group; use of personality assessment instruments that were either not validated or validated only in psychiatric samples; and failure to consider the effects of age, gender, and coexisting anxiety and mood disorders.

The few population-based studies suggest that those with migraine exhibited significantly greater scores for neuroticism as compared with controls [28–32]. However, the neuroticism scores are not specific and may be more reflective of the presence of chronic pain. Results of smaller, clinical studies using the Minnesota Multiphasic Personality Inventory (MMPI) [32] confirm the data obtained in the general population: the 'neurotic triad' scores (hypochondria, depression, hysteria) are higher in headache patients, but still do not reach the pathological threshold.

Mechanisms of migraine comorbidity with psychiatric disorders

There are three basic mechanisms that could underlie psychiatric comorbidity with migraine:
1 Psychiatric disorders are a causal factor in the development of migraine.
2 Migraine is a causal factor in the development of psychiatric disorders (e.g., repeated and intense pain may lead to anticipating anxiety, perceived loss of control and other behavioral or cognitive risk factors for psychiatric syndromes).
3 A common shared etiological factor may explain the co-occurrence of both syndromes (e.g., a common genetic factor may result in abnormalities in neurotransmission, hormone regulation or other biological abnormalities) [33,34].

Table 1.1 Lifetime comorbidity of migraine and psychiatric disorders in population-based studies.

	Risk-ratio and confidence interval				
	Merikangas et al. 1990	Breslau et al. 1991	Swartz et al. 2000	Jette et al. 2008	Saunders et al. 2008
Comorbid disorder					
Major depressive disorder	2.2 (1.1–4.8)	4.3 (3.0–6.9)	3.2 (2.0–4.8)	2.3 (1.9–2.8)	3.5 (2.6–4.6)
Bipolar I and II	2.9 (1.1–8.6)	NS	7.3 (2.2–24.6)	3.7 (2.7–5.0)	3.9 (2.3–6.5)
Obsessive compulsive disorder	1.0 NS	5.1 (2.3–11.2)	NS	—	—
Generalized anxiety disorder	3.3	5.7 (2.7–12.1)	NS		2.5 (1.6–4.0)
Panic disorder	5.3			2.8 (2.2–3.6)	3.6 (2.4–5.2)
Social phobia	3.4 (1.1–10.9)	2.6 (1.5–3.3)	1.6 (1.3–2.2)	2.3 (1.9–2.9)	2.4 (1.8–2.3)
Nicotine dependence	—	2.2 (1.5–3.3)	—	—	4.6 (1.4–11.1)
Substance-related disorders	—	2.2 (1.5–3.3)	NS	1.0 (NS)	1.6 (0.9–2.9) NS
Any mental disorder	3.3 (0.8–13.8)	6.6 (3.2–13.9)	5.1 (2.6–9.8)	3.1 (2.4–4.1)	3.7 (2.2–6.2)

NS, non-significant.

Attempts to disentangle these three possible mechanisms have focused on assessing the order of onset of these conditions using longitudinal study designs, by measuring the change in severity of one disorder in the presence of comorbidity, and by examining the co-transmission of these disorders within families.

Few studies have assessed the order of onset of psychiatric disorders and migraine, and those available fail to provide a clear picture of the association amongst these conditions. Results from the Zurich Cohort Study show that anxiety disorders, including social phobia, simple phobia, agoraphobia, generalized anxiety disorder (GAD) and panic precede the onset of migraine headaches, which in turn precede the onset of affective disorders [5,35]. Similar results were obtained from the Dunedin Multidisciplinary Health and Development Study, which reported that individuals with migraine at age 26 had increased odds of an anxiety disorder at age 18 or 21 years [36]. Although results from the 13-year prospective follow-up of the Epidemiologic Catchment Area Study confirmed that a history of phobic disorder was predictive of the onset of migraine [9], they did not find that the onset of panic disorder systematically preceded that of migraine. In 1993, Breslau and Davis [2] found that migraine was also related to the subsequent onset of both major depression and panic disorder. Therefore, although the current evidence regarding order of onset suggests that migraine, anxiety and depressive disorders may co-occur because of common underlying etiologic factors, additional prospective research is necessary to obtain more conclusive evidence.

Findings of a linear relationship between headache frequency and the rate of comorbidity in the general population [11], and the association between the number of days with migraine and intensity of emotional distress [24] support the hypothesis of a common underlying aetiology between emotional disorders and migraine. However, the specific risk factors have not yet been identified [5,37,38]. Possible mechanisms include alterations in monoamine systems or channelopathies [39], which have been considered in the pathogenesis of both migraine [20] and mood disorders [40]. Further research is needed to identify these potential pathways to migraine and mood/anxiety disorders.

Impact of psychiatric comorbidity on migraine

Several studies have investigated the clinical consequences of psychiatric comorbidity in individuals with migraine. The results of two French studies are shown in Figures 1.1–1.3. FRAMIG (Figures 1.1 and 1.2) was a nationwide, population-based postal survey, the objectives of which were to analyze the relationship between disability, quality of life and psychiatric comorbidity in migraine sufferers [24]. The objectives of the SMILE study (Figure 1.3) were to assess anxiety, stress, depression, functional impact and coping behaviors in 5417 consulting migraine patients [41]. Migraine patients with elevated anxiety and depression scores have worse quality of life than those patients without psychiatric comorbidity (Figure 1.1) [(10,16,21,24]. Similarly, psychiatric comorbidity in migraine patients is associated with increased disability

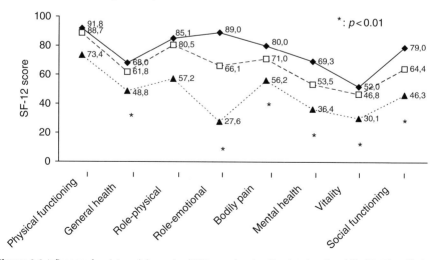

Figure 1.1 Influence of anxiety and depression (HAD scores) on health-related quality of life (SF-12) profile in FRAMIG study (population-based sample of migraine subjects). Migraine subjects with anxiety and those with both anxiety and depression differed significantly ($p < 0.01$) from migraine subjects with neither anxiety nor depression on all eight SF-12 dimensions except for physical functioning and role-physical.

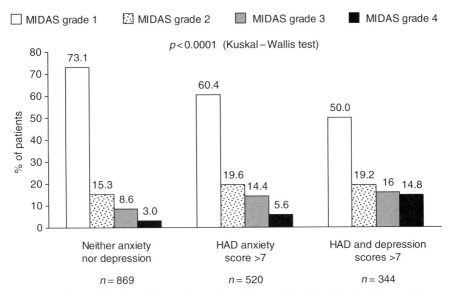

Figure 1.2 Influence of anxiety and depression (HAD scores) on migraine-related disability (MIDAS grade) in FRAMIG study (population-based subject sample).

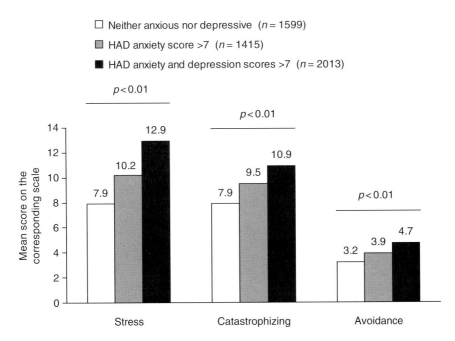

Figure 1.3 Effect of anxiety and depression (HAD scale) on perceived stress, catastrophizing and avoidance in SMILE study (sample of primary-care consulting migraine patients). Stress evaluated using the abridged form (PSS4) of the original Perceived Stress Scale questionnaire [59]; catastrophizing evaluated using the catastrophizing subscale of the Coping Strategies Questionnaire (CSQ) [60]; avoidance evaluated using the behavioral disengagement subscale of the brief version of the COPE inventory [61,62].

(as measured by the MIDAS score) (Figure 1.2) [24,41], and with an increase in direct costs related to migraine (such as those attributable to medications and health services) [42]. Moreover, a study by Radat et al. [41] indicates that perceived stress, catastrophizing and avoidance behaviors are more pronounced in migraine patients with elevated anxiety and depression scores than in migraine patients without psychiatric comorbidity (Figure 1.3). Finally, psychiatric comorbidity is associated with a greater number of days with migraine attacks, a greater number of days using acute antimigraine medications [41], and with poorer satisfaction with the efficacy of acute treatments [24]. This is in agreement with the finding that comorbidity with anxiety and depression is greater in patients with chronic migraine and up to four times greater in patients with MOH evolving from migraine than in those with episodic migraine [43,27]. Comorbidity with anxiety and depression, therefore, appears to be associated with both chronicity and analgesic abuse. These findings underscore the importance of identifying migraine patients suffering from psychiatric comorbidity as they are likely to display more severe symptoms, greater disability and report a worse quality of life [16].

Management

The strong association of migraine with both depression and anxiety should be considered in the treatment of individuals with migraine [44]. Systematic evaluation of the lifetime history of both depression and anxiety is necessary for determining optimal treatment strategies. Clinicians should systematically consider comorbid anxiety and mood disorders in selecting treatment options for people with migraine. Jette et al. [15] found that people from the general population with both a mental disorder and migraine were significantly more likely to take an antidepressant than those with either depression or anxiety alone or migraine alone. In general, comorbid depression and anxiety are more relevant for the selection of a migraine prophylaxis than for that of an acute antimigraine treatment. The use of prophylactic medications with side effects of lassitude, fatigue or depression should be avoided, if possible. If not, careful clinical evaluation of the above-cited manifestations of depression, including anergia, hypersomnia and irritability, should be monitored. Additionally, in patients with medication overuse headache evolving from episodic migraine, it is critical to evaluate the potential for dependence on acute antimigraine drugs, which would impose specific management of the behavior underlying drug consumption.

Regarding pharmacological options for treatment, the major classes of drugs that have been investigated in the prophylaxis of migraine include the β-adrenergic blocking agents, antidepressants, anticonvulsants, calcium channel blockers and aspirin [44]. The beta-blockers have been the most widely prescribed class of drugs for migraine prophylaxis; however, clinicians should be particularly cautious in prescribing this class of drugs to individuals with a history of depression, since the beta-blockers are associated with the development of anhedonia, irritability and lassitude, which may occur after many months on any of these agents. In contrast, patients with high levels of autonomic anxiety may actually benefit from this class of drugs.

The tricyclic antidepressants have been well-established as prophylactic agents for migraine; however, the side effects of amitriptyline include sedation and weight gain. Secondary amines (e.g., nortriptyline and desipramine) appear to be efficacious in the treatment of depression, and have fewer side effects than do the parent tertiary amines (e.g., amitriptyline, imipramine). Conversely, the selective serotonin reuptake inhibitors (SSRIs) have not demonstrated efficacy in migraine. In fact, some patients complain of headache as a secondary effect of the latter class of drugs [45]. Introducing the SSRI very slowly reduces this inconvenience. The combination of these drugs with triptans poses a theoretical risk of inducing serotoninergic syndromes. In practice, the risk appears extremely low and related to the addition of a third serotoninergic drug or the use of elevated doses [46]. In the future, dual serotonin and norepinephrine (noradrenaline) reuptake inhibitors may be established as effective drugs for the preventive treatment of migraine in patients with anxious and depressive disorders [47–49].

The monoamine oxidase inhibitors (MAOIs), which have been demonstrated to be superior to other classes of antidepressants in the management of depression with atypical features [50], have also been reported to be efficacious in the treatment of migraine headache [51,52]. However, this class of drugs should be reserved for people with frequent and severe migraine accompanied by atypical depression and anxiety disorders.

Antiepileptic drugs such as valproate and, to a lesser extent, topiramate, may be useful for mood regulation in patients with bipolar mood disorders or, for divalproate specifically, the treatment of bipolar depression [53]. Worthy of note is that depression can be an adverse effect of topiramate. Nevertheless, bipolarity should be carefully assessed in depressed patients and these drugs preferentially given to bipolar subjects over antidepressants since antidepressants can precipitate a mood switch.

There has been substantial research on the use of behavioral treatments including biofeedback, relaxation training, and cognitive-behavioral therapy for migraine prevention. Alternative treatments of relaxation (and/or biofeedback) and cognitive-behavioral therapy have demonstrated their efficacy in the prophylactic treatment of migraine [54–56] but overall their efficacy is below that of pharmacological treatments. They can, however, be effectively associated with the latter, in particular in stress-sensitive subjects. The efficacy of interpersonal and cognitive therapy for the treatment of acute episodes of depression may also extend to the treatment of depression in the context of migraine. These approaches may be particularly useful for migraine patients with anxious anticipation of attacks, which can lead to MOH, as well as those patients for whom stress is a predominant trigger factor of attacks [57]. Stress perception and dysfunctional coping strategies such as catastrophizing and avoidance can be targeted by psychotherapeutic interventions [58].

Case report: treatment approach

In a first step, ambulatory withdrawal was proposed to Miss E. after two consultations with center physicians (a neurologist and a psychiatrist) and an interview with the nurse. These interviews were intended to assess the current medical condition, to make treatment objectives clear for the patient and to initiate therapeutic education. In particular, we educated the patient in the keeping of a headache diary, with a record of intakes of acute antimigraine treatments. During the withdrawal period, the patient was asked to take no more than two tablets per week of frovatriptan (the acute treatment was changed) and we initiated a preventive treatment with valproate. The selection of this drug was based on the possibility that the patient's mood disorder pertained to the bipolar spectrum. Withdrawal headaches staggered over the first five days and were bravely endured by the patient. To help her, we proposed psychological support and relaxation sessions. Relaxation therapy was proposed on the basis of one session per week during the first two months, and we advised the patient to complement them with a stress management therapy. Evolution was favorable, both concerning migraine as well as mood.

Conclusion

There is substantial evidence for the association of migraine with psychiatric disorders. This review of the literature suggests the following:

1 Individuals with migraine show increased odds of developing depressive disorders or anxiety disorders, especially panic attacks, generalized anxiety and phobic disorders, as well as bipolar mood disorders.
2 The mechanisms of comorbidity likely comprise both common risk factors and causal links. Repercussions of comorbidity include alterations in onset, course and severity of migraine; greater deterioration of quality of life; and increase in the frequency of intake of antimigraine drugs, which increases the probability that episodic migraine will evolve to MOH. The management proposed to the patient will then take this aspect into account.
3 Potential treatments for migraine accompanied by depression include antidepressants and other mood regulators; they may simultaneously lead to remission of symptoms of migraine and co-occurring depression, anxiety and bipolar mood disorders.

References

1 Breslau N, Davis GC, Andreski P. Migraine, psychiatric disorders, and suicide attempts: an epidemiologic study of young adults. Psychiat Res 1991; 37:11–23.
2 Breslau N, Davis GC. Migraine, physical health and psychiatric disorder: a prospective epidemiologic study in young adults. J Psychiatr Res 1993;27:211–21.

Psychiatric Comorbidity in Migraine   **11**

3 Breslau N, Davis GC, Schultz LR, Peterson EL. Joint 1994 Wolff Award Presentation. Migraine and major depression. Headache 1994;34:387–93.

4 Breslau N, Schultz LR, Stewart WF, Lipton RB, Lucia VC, Welch KMA. Headache and major depression. Is the association specific to migraine? Neurology 2000;54:308–13.

5 Merikangas KR, Merikangas JR, Angst J. Headache syndromes and psychiatric disorders: association and familial transmission. J Psychiatr Res 1993;27:197–210.

6 Merikangas KR. Psychopathology and headache syndromes in the community. Headache 1994;34:S17–S26.

7 Devlen J. Anxiety and depression in migraine. J Royal Soc Med 1994,87:338–41.

8 Wang SJ, Liu HC, Fuh JL, Wang PN, Lu SR. Comorbidity of headache and depression in the elderly. Pain 1999;82:239–43.

9 Swartz KL, Pratt LA, Armenian HK, Lee LC, Eaton WW. Mental disorders and the incidence of migraine headaches in a community sample. Arch Gen Psychiatry 2000;57:945–50.

10 Lipton RB, Hamelsky SW, Kolodner KB, Steiner TJ, Stewart WF. Migraine, quality of life, and depression: a population-based case-control study. Neurology 2000;55:629–35.

11 Zwart JA, Dyb G, Hagen K, et al. Depression and anxiety disorders associated with headache frequency. The Nord-Trøndelag Health Study. Eur J Neurol 2003;10:147–52.

12 McWilliams LA, Goodwin RD, Cox BJ. Depression and anxiety associated with three pain conditions: results from a nationally representative sample. Pain 2004;111:77–83.

13 Patel NV, Bigal ME, Kolodner KB, Leotta C, Lafata JE, Lipton RB. Prevalence and impact of migraine and probable migraine in a health plan. Neurology 2004;63:1432–8.

14 Oedegaard KJ, Neckelmann D, Mykletun A, et al. Migraine with and without aura: association with depression and anxiety disorder in a population-based study. The HUNT Study. Cephalalgia 2006;26:1–6.

15 Jette N, Patten S, William J, Becker W, Siebe S. Comorbidity of migraine and psychiatric disorders: A national population-based study. Headache 2008;48:501–16.

16 Saunders K, Merikangas K, Low NC, Von Korff M, Kessler RC. Impact of comorbidity on headache-related disability. Neurology 2008;70:538–47.

17 Marazziti D, Toni C, Pedri S, et al. Headache, panic disorder and depression: comorbidity or a spectrum? Neuropsychobiology 1995;31:125–9.

18 Juang KD, Wang SJ, Fuh JL, Lu SR, Su TP. Comorbidity of depressive and anxiety disorders in chronic daily headache and its subtypes. Headache 2000;40:818–23.

19 Wang S-J. Migraine and suicide. Expert Rev Neurotherapeutics 2007;7:1069–71.

20 Mahmood T, Romans S, Silverstone T. Prevalence of migraine in bipolar disorder. J Affect Disord 1999;52:239–41.

21 Fasmer OB. The prevalence of migraine in patients with bipolar and unipolar affective disorders. Cephalalgia 2001;21:894–9.

22 McIntyre RS, Konarski JZ, Wilkins K, Bouffard B, Soczynska JK, Kennedy SH. The prevalence and impact of migraine headache in bipolar disorder: results from the Canadian Community Health Survey. Headache 2006;46:973–82.

23 Breslau N, Schultz LR, Stewart WF, Lipton R, Welch KM. Headache types and panic disorder: directionality and specificity. Neurology 2001;56:350–4.

24 Lantéri-Minet M, Radat F, Chautard MH, Lucas C. Anxiety and depression associated with migraine: influence on migraine subjects' disability and quality of life, and acute migraine management. Pain 2005;118:319–26.

25 Radat F, Creac'h C, Guégan-Massardier E, et al. Behavioral dependence in patients with medication overuse headache: a cross-sectional study in consulting patients using the DSM-IV criteria. Headache 2008;48:1026–36.

26 Fuh JL, Wang SJ, Lu SR, Juang KD. Does medication overuse headache represent a behavior of dependence? Pain 2005;119:49–55.

27 Radat F, Creac'h C, Swendsen JD, et al. From migraine to headache induced by chronic substance use: the role of psychiatric co-morbidity. Cephalalgia 2005;25:519–22.

28 Merikangas KR, Stevens DE, Angst J. Headache and personality: Results of a community sample of young adults. J Psychiatr Res 1993;27:187–96.

29 Henryk-Gutt R, Rees WL. Psychological aspects of migraine. J Psychosom Res 1973;17:141–53.

30 Brandt J, Celentano D, Stewart W, Linet M, Folstein MF. Personality and emotional disorder in a community sample of migraine headache sufferers. Am J Psychiatry 1990;147:303–8.

31 Rasmussen BK. Migraine and tension-type headache in a general population: psychosocial factors. Int J Epidemiol 1992;21:1138–43.

32 Breslau N, Andreski P. Migraine, personality and psychiatric comorbidity. Headache 1995;35:382–6.

33 Silberstein SD, Lipton RB, Breslau N. Migraine: association with personality characteristics and psychopathology. Cephalalgia 1995;15:358–69.

34 Wittchen HU. Critical issues in the evaluation of comorbidity of psychiatric disorders. Br J Psychiatry Suppl 1996;30:9–16.

35 Merikangas KR, Angst J, Isler H. Migraine and psychopathology. Results of the Zurich cohort study of young adults. Arch Gen Psychiatry 1990;47:849–53.

36 Waldie KE, Poulton R. Physical and psychological correlates of primary headache in young adulthood: a 26-year longitudinal study. J Neurol Neurosurg Psychiatry 2002;72:86–92.

37 Merikangas KR, Risch NJ, Merikangas JR, Weissman MM, Kidd KK. Migraine and depression: association and familial transmission. J Psychiatr Res 1988;22:119–29.

38 Franchini L, Bongiorno F, Dotoli D, Rainero I, Pinessi L, Smeraldi E. Migraine headache and mood disorders: a descriptive study in an outpatient psychiatric population. J Affect Disord 2004;81:157–60.

39 Lea RA, Curtain RP, Hutchins C, Brimage PJ, Grilliths LR. Investigation of the CACNA1A gene as a candidate for typical migraine susceptibility. Am J Med Genet 2001;105,8:707–12

40 Shiah IS, Ko HC, Lee JF, Lur B. Platelet 5-HT and plasma MHPG levels in patients with bipolar I and bipolar II depressions and normal controls. J. Affect Disord 1999;52:101–10.

41 Radat F, Mekies C, Géraud G, et al. Anxiety, stress and coping behaviours in primary care migraine patients: results of SMILE study. Cephalalgia 2008;28:1115–25.

42 Pesa J, Lage MJ. The medical costs of migraine and comorbid anxiety and depression. Headache 2004;44:562–70.

43 Radat F, Sakh D, Lutz G, El Amrani M, Ferreri M, Bousser MG. Psychiatric comorbidity is related to headache induced by chronic substance use in migraineurs. Headache 1999;39:477–80.

44 Merikangas JR, Merikangas KR, Khoromi S. Neuropsychiatric aspects of headaches. In: Sadock BJ, Sadock VA, Ruiz P (eds) Comprehensive Textbook of Psychiatry, 9th edn. Wolters Kluwer, 2007; Chap. 2.11.

45 Moja PL, Cusi C, Sterzi RR, Canepari C. Selective serotonin re-uptake inhibitors (SSRIs) for preventing migraine and tension-type headaches. Cochrane Db Syst Rev 2005;20(3):CD002919.

46 Shapiro RE, Tepper SJ. The serotonin syndrome, triptans, and the potential for drug–drug interactions. Headache 2007;47:266–9.

47 Adelman LC, Adelman JU, Von Seggern R, Mannix LK. Venlafaxine extended release (XR) for the prophylaxis of migraine and tension-type headache: a retrospective study in a clinical setting. Headache 2000;40:572–80.

48 Bulut S, Berilgen MS, Baran A, Tekatas A, Atmaca M, Mungen B. Venlafaxine versus amitriptyline in the prophylactic treatment of migraine: randomized, double-blind, crossover study. Clin Neurol Neurosurg 2004;107:44–8.

49 Ozyalcin SN, Talu GK, Kiziltan E, Yucel B, Ertas M, Disci R. The efficacy and safety of venlafaxine in the prophylaxis of migraine. Headache 2005;45:144–52.

50 Stewart JW. Treating depression with atypical features. J Clin Psychiatry 2007;68(Suppl. 3):25–9.

51 Merikangas KR, Merikangas JR. Combination monoamine oxidase inhibitor and B-blocker treatment of migraine, with anxiety and depression. Biol Psychiatry 1995;38:603–10.

52 Raskin NH. Headache, 2nd edn. New York: Churchill Livingstone, 1988.

53 Goodwin FK, Jamison KR. Manic Depressive Illness. Oxford: Oxford University Press, 2007.

54 Holroyd KA, Penzien DB. Psychosocial interventions in the management of recurrent headache disorders. 1: Overview and effectiveness. Behavioral Med 1994;20:53–63.

55 Campbell JK, Penzien DB, Wall EM. Evidence-based Guidelines for Migraine Headache: Behavioral and Physical Treatments. St Paul: American Academy of Neurology, 2000.

56 Rains JC, Penzien DB, McCrory DC, Gray RN. Behavioral headache treatment: history, review of the empirical literature, and methodological critique. Headache 2005;45(Suppl. 2):92–109.

57 Lipchik GL, Smitherman TA, Penzien DB, Holroyd KA. Basic principles and techniques of cognitive-behavioral therapies for comorbid psychiatric symptoms among headache patients. Headache 2006;46(Suppl. 3):119–32.

58 Thorn BE, Pence LB, Ward LC, et al. A randomized clinical trial of targeted cognitive behavioral treatment to reduce catastrophizing in chronic headache sufferers. J Pain 2007;8:938–49.

59 Cohen S, Kamarck T, Mermelstein R. A global measure of perceived stress. J Health Soc Behav 1983;24:385–96.

60 Rosenstiel AK, Keefe FJ. The use of coping strategies in chronic low back pain patients: relationship to patient characteristics and current adjustment. Pain 1983;17:33–44.

61 Carver CS. You want to measure coping but your protocol's too long: consider the brief COPE. Int J Behav Med 1997;4:92–100.

62 Müller L, Spitz E. Multidimensional assessment of coping: validation of the Brief COPE among the French population. Encephale 2003;29:507–18.

2 Migraine and Stroke

Tobias Kurth[1] and Hans-Christoph Diener[2]

[1] Inserm Unit 708-Neuroepidemiology and University Pierre et Marie Curie, Paris, France; Division of Preventive Medicine, Brigham and Women's Hospital, Harvard Medical School and Department of Epidemiology, Harvard School of Public Health, Boston, MA, USA
[2] Department of Neurology, University of Duisburg-Essen, Essen, Germany

Introduction

Migraine and stroke are very common diseases, although their age- and sex-specific occurrences are very different. Migraine is a disease of younger individuals, mostly women [1], whereas the incidence of stroke increases exponentially after the age of 65 and is more common in men [2]. A link between these two diseases seems at first glance unlikely. However, migraine and stroke share common clinical features, and many studies have suggested a close link [3].

Dysfunction of brain cells and arteries is a major component of migraine pathophysiology [4,5]. The vascular dysfunction of cerebral arteries during the migraine attack has led to the hypothesis that migraine may be a risk factor for ischemic stroke. Indeed, several case-control studies and three prospective cohort studies found increased risk of ischemic stroke, in particular among young women with migraine with aura [6–11]. A systematic meta-analysis of observational studies showed that the risk of ischemic stroke was significantly increased among all migraineurs but magnified for those with migraine aura [12]. In addition, migraine has been associated with silent brain lesions, mostly in the white matter [13,14]. However, because migraine is very prevalent in age groups in which a stroke event is very rare, the absolute risk of stroke for migraine patients is low [10,15], and it seems plausible that in addition to migraine, other factors need to be present to substantially increase the risk of ischemic stroke. Although some studies found increased risk for women with migraine who smoke or use oral contraceptives, overall it remains unclear which migraine patients are at particular risk of experiencing a stroke.

This chapter aims to provide an overview of the association between migraine and ischemic stroke, discuss potential biological mechanisms and factors associated with particular increased risk, and to illustrate the potential consequences for the care of migraine patients.

Comorbidity in Migraine, First Edition. Edited by J. Schoenen, D. W. Dodick and P. S. Sándor.

Epidemiology

The association between migraine and stroke has emerged over the last decades, and several retrospective case-control [6,7,15–21], prospective [9–11], and cross-sectional cohort studies [22], as well as studies using data from stroke registries [23,24] have been published on this topic. The case-control studies found increased risk of ischemic stroke among women less than 45 years of age who reported a history of migraine with aura [7,15,20], with risk estimates ranging from 3.8 [7] to 8.4 [20], and additional case-control studies [6,17] found increased risk for migraineurs with aura among both genders. Only in one case-control study was migraine without aura associated with increased risk of ischemic stroke [15]. The association between migraine and hemorrhagic stroke was only evaluated in one case-control study [7], which found increased risk for those with a family history of migraine [relative risk (RR) = 2.30; 95% confidence interval (CI) = 1.35–3.90] and also suggested there might be an increased risk among participants with migraine without aura (RR = 1.84; 95% CI = 0.77–4.39). In another case-control study, the association between migraine and hemorrhagic stroke produced conflicting results, since it was dependent on the control selection [25]. When the interaction between migraine and other risk factors for stroke was evaluated, the risk was more than tripled by smoking (RR = 10) [15] and quadrupled by oral contraceptive use (RR = 13.9–16.9) [7,15]. The combination of migraine, oral contraceptives and smoking further increases the risk [26].

A meta-analysis of 11 case-control and three cohort studies published before 2004 suggested that the risk of stroke is increased in people with migraine (pooled RR = 2.16; 95% CI = 1.89–2.48). This risk was highest among patients with migraine with aura (RR = 2.27; 95% CI = 1.61–3.19) but also apparent among those migraineurs without aura (RR = 1.83; 95% CI = 1.06–3.15). The risk was markedly increased for women taking oral contraceptives (RR = 8.72; 95% CI = 5.05–15.05) [12].

Two large-scale prospective cohort studies and one population-based case-control study have been published that support the results of the meta-analysis but provide evidence that the association between migraine and stroke is limited to migraineurs with aura. The first prospective study used data from the Women's Health Study, which included over 39,000 apparently healthy women aged 45 years or older [10]. This study found a 1.7-fold increased risk for ischemic stroke (RR = 1.71; 95% CI = 1.11–2.66) for women who reported migraine with aura when compared to women without migraine. This risk was stronger in those who were 45 to 55 years of age (RR = 2.25; 95% CI = 1.30–3.91) and was not seen in the older age group. Migraine without aura was not associated with an increased risk of ischemic stroke. Furthermore, there was no association between any migraine type and hemorrhagic stroke [10]. A recent update from this study cohort evaluated the impact of migraine attack frequency of <monthly, monthly, or ≥ weekly on risk of subsequent cardiovascular disease (CVD) [27]. The association between migraine attack frequency and ischemic

stroke was J-shaped. Compared with women without migraine, the RRs (95% CIs) for ischemic stroke were 1.90 (1.18–3.08) for women with migraine with aura with a migraine attack frequency <monthly and 4.25 (1.36–13.29) for a migraine frequency of ≥ weekly.

The second prospective study used data from the Atherosclerosis Risk in Communities Study and included over 12,000 men and women mostly aged 55 and older [11]. The study evaluated the migraine–stroke association in different time windows (i.e., retrospective and prospective). The strict prospective evaluation (i.e., the migraine assessment preceded the stroke event) showed a 1.8-fold increased risk of ischemic stroke (RR = 1.84; 95% CI = 0.89–3.82) for migraineurs with aura when compared to participants without migraine. The fact that the risk estimates did not reach statistical significance may be due to the specific migraine and aura classification of that study [28]. This study found no further effect modification by age, and the migraine–stroke association persisted after controlling for a large number of traditional stroke risk factors. The results of these prospective studies suggest that the migraine–stroke association may not be limited to individuals under the age of 45.

The Stroke Prevention in Young Women Study matched 386 women age 15–49 with first ischemic stroke with 614 age- and ethnicity-matched controls [26]. Subjects were classified as having no headache, probable migraine without visual symptoms, and probable migraine with visual symptoms. Compared with women without headache, those who reported probable migraine with visual symptoms had a 1.5-fold increased risk of ischemic stroke (RR = 1.5; 95% CI = 1.1–2.0), which attenuated after control for stroke risk factors. This risk further increased for women who reported a probable migraine frequency of at least 12 per year (RR = 2.3; 95% CI = 1.5–3.5) and for those who had begun having migraines during the prior year (RR = 6.7; 95% CI = 2.3–19.2). Women with probable migraine without visual symptoms were not at increased risk for ischemic stroke. When effect modification by smoking and oral contraceptive use was considered, neither factor by itself substantially increased the risk of ischemic stroke among women with probable headache with aura. However, when the combination of smoking and oral contraceptive use was taken into account, the risk of ischemic stroke was seven-fold increased when compared with women without probable migraine. When compared with women without probable migraine who did not smoke and who did not use oral contraceptive, this risk was even further increased to 10-fold [26].

A large cross-sectional study using a nationwide inpatient sample from the USA evaluated the association of migraine with ischemic events during pregnancy [29]. Diagnoses of migraine and outcome events were identified by ICD-9 (International Classification of Diseases, 9th revision) codes. Of over 18 million pregnancy-related discharges, 33,956 migraine codes were identified. Women with migraine codes were at substantially increased risk of stroke (RR = 15.05; 95% CI = 8.26–27.4), which was particularly strong for ischemic stroke (RR = 30.7; 95% CI = 17.4–34.1) but also apparent for intracerebral hemorrhage (RR = 9.1; 95% CI = 3.0–27.8). The study further found a strong association with other ischemic events.

While the cross-sectional nature of the study as well as potential coding biases should signal caution about interpretation of the study, migraine during pregnancy may be a marker for women at increased risk for vascular events.

In summary, there is good epidemiologic evidence that migraine with aura is associated with an increased risk of ischemic stroke, which appears to be stronger among the young but may persist in the elderly. Prospective data do not support an association between migraine without aura and ischemic stroke. There is currently little evidence that migraine increases the risk of hemorrhagic stroke.

Pathophysiology

The mechanisms by which migraine may increase the risk of ischemic stroke remain unclear but are likely complex. Several potential mechanisms can be envisioned: (i) migraine may directly cause an ischemic stroke (i.e., a migrainous infarct); (ii) migraine pathophysiology interferes with existing local vascular pathologies and both jointly increase the risk of stroke outside of a migraine attack; (iii) migraine is associated with an increased prevalence of vascular risk factors, congenital heart defects, or other risk factors for stroke; (iv) migraine-specific treatments; and (v) migraine and ischemic stroke are linked via genetic factors.

Migrainous infarction

The second International Classification of Headache Disorders (ICHD-2) defines a migrainous infarction as one or more aura symptoms associated with an ischemic brain lesion in an appropriate territory demonstrated by neuroimaging. This ischemic brain lesion must occur in conjunction with a migraine attack in a patient with migraine with aura, which is typical of previous attacks except that one or more aura symptoms persists for more than 60 minutes. Other causes for ischemia have to be ruled out [30]. There are insufficient data on the incidence of migrainous infarction based on the strict ICHD-2 definition. Prior to the ICHD-2, a study from the UK found seven (3%) migrainous infarcts out of 244 first ischemic strokes, albeit with little diagnostic validation [31]. In other studies, migrainous infarcts accounted for 0.5–1.5% of all ischemic strokes, with a much higher proportion in younger patients (~12%) [23,32–34]. This mechanism may also be the cause of silent cerebral infarctions and white matter lesions in migraine patients, which is covered in Chapter 3. However, most ischemic strokes among migraine patients occur between attacks and not during or shortly after a migraine attack with aura [15,16]; therefore, a migrainous infarction is unlikely to explain the overall migraine–stroke association.

Interaction with other pathologies

It is also possible that migraine pathophysiology, which during aura is associated with reductions in cerebral blood flow, augments existing vascular pathologies, and both jointly increase the risk of ischemic vascular events. In the face of concomitant local vascular damage or coexisting vascular risk factors influencing the tendency for local thrombosis, it is conceivable that permanent ischemic events may occur. Another potential mechanism involves artery dissection, with some studies suggesting mostly dissections in the cervical arteries [35–37]. The associated relative risk values of these case-control studies varied from 3.6 [36] to 7.4 [37]. Patients with a suspected migrainous infarct should be investigated for potential artery dissections.

Postmenopausal hormone replacement has been associated with both migraine [38] and ischemic stroke [39], making involvement of female hormones a plausible mechanism underlying the relationship between migraine and ischemic stroke. However, this mechanism seems rather unlikely to explain the association between migraine and stroke since hormones play a role not only in migraineurs with aura but also among those without aura, and it is particularly migraine with aura that is associated with increased risk of stroke.

In some patients, migraine and ischemic stroke occur commonly as part of distinct disorders. These include cerebral autosomal dominant arteriopathy with subcortical infarcts and leukoencephalopathy (CADASIL) [40,41]; mitochondrial myopathy, encephalopathy, lactacidosis and stroke (MELAS) [42]; and autosomal dominant vascular retinopathy, migraine and Raynaud phenomenon [3,43]. These, however, are distinct diseases affecting only very few migraine patients and are thus not the explanation of the overall migraine–stroke association.

The association between migraine and stroke is complex and potentially bidirectional [3,28], and migraine attacks can be induced by cerebral ischemia [44]. Sometimes, ischemic strokes can present with migraine attacks [45–47]. In animal studies, cerebral ischemia can induce cortical spreading depression [48]. This has implications for studies that evaluate whether migraine is a risk factor for stroke.

Migraine and cardiovascular risk factors

Some studies have suggested that migraine is more frequent among individuals with normal or lower blood pressure [49,50]. However, in large population-based studies, migraine was associated with a higher prevalence of hypertension [51,52]. The Genetic Epidemiology of Migraine study [52] found that compared to controls, migraineurs are more likely to smoke and are more likely to have a parental history of early myocardial infarction. The study also found that migraineurs with aura are more likely to have an unfavorable cholesterol profile, elevated blood pressure, report a history of early-onset coronary heart disease or stroke, and have a two-fold increased risk of a high Framingham-risk score-predicted 10-year risk of coronary heart disease even after adjusting for age [52,53]. Furthermore, recent studies have linked migraine frequency and severity with increased body mass index [54,55]. Thus, one could speculate that the coexistence of vascular risk factors plays a role in the migraine–stroke association. In addition, recent data suggest that migraine with aura is also a marker for increased risk of any ischemic vascular events, including myocardial infarction and cardiovascular death [56–58], an association discussed in detail in Chapter 3.

However, in most studies that have evaluated the migraine–stroke association, the estimated RR was not attenuated after controlling for cardiovascular risk factors [10,11,15,22]. In addition, studies have suggested that the increased risk of ischemic stroke is more apparent among individuals without cardiovascular risk factors [6,10,24,55], with the exception of smoking and/or oral contraceptive use or their combination [26]. This is supported by recent results from the Women's Health Study, indicating that the association between migraine with aura and ischemic stroke is only apparent among women with a low Framingham risk score for coronary heart disease (RR = 3.88; 95% CI = 1.87–8.08) [59]. This interesting observation may also explain why the association between migraine and stroke diminishes with increasing age in most studies: other major risk factors for ischemic stroke, such as hypertension and diabetes, acquire greater importance with increasing age or interact with the mechanism by which migraine may lead to stroke. This would result in a relatively reduced influence of migraine as a risk factor for ischemic stroke with increasing age. However, the diminishing association between migraine and stroke in the elderly may also be related to a migraine-specific mechanism. It is further interesting that the association between migraine with aura and myocardial infarction shows a diametric association pattern, indicating that only the high-vascular-risk group among migraineurs with aura is at risk [59].

Patent foramen ovale

Patent foramen ovale (PFO) is an often asymptomatic condition that is present in approximately 25% of the general population. Several clinic-based case-control studies have suggested that PFO is more common among individuals with migraine with aura and that migraine with aura is more common among individuals with PFO [60–64]. This has led to speculation that PFO might be causally linked with migraine with aura, and that this link is the reason for the observed increased risk of ischemic stroke among migraineurs with aura. Specifically, it has been suggested that the right-to-left shunt may serve as a conduit for the passage of particulate or humoral factors from the venous to arterial circulation, which then, in a predisposed individual with migraine, could serve to trigger an attack. It can be envisioned that such a mechanism either induces cortical spreading depression [5] or triggers another mechanism leading to migraine with aura [3,63]. However, results from a population-based case-control study did not indicate significant differences in stroke risk for migraineurs with and without aura according to PFO status [26]. Despite low-grade evidence linking migraine with PFO [65] and recent population-based data showing no association between migraine and PFO [66], this association has stimulated immense interest, and several observational studies as well as randomized clinical trials have been initiated investigating whether PFO closure leads to reduced migraine attack frequency and migraine burden. However, observation studies indicating potentially beneficial results [63] were in contrast to the negative results of the Migraine Intervention with STARFlex© Technology (MIST) trial. Other trials, such as MIST II, have meanwhile been stopped due to low enrollment rates. Further details on the association between PFO and migraine are discussed in Chapter 4.

Genetic polymorphisms

The familial hemiplegic form of migraine is also an autosomal dominant disorder. The gene has been mapped to chromosome 19p3 in about two-thirds of cases [67,68]. Another gene for the familial hemiplegic migraine has been identified on chromosome 1q21–23 [69]. However, genetic aspects underlying the common forms of migraine have not been established. Because of the broad clinical spectrum of migraine, the interaction of several polymorphisms is likely to determine the manifestation and severity of migraine, and the effect of a single genetic mutation is expected to be small. Migraine, in particular migraine with aura, has been associated with the *MTHFR C677T* genotype in some [70,71] but not all studies [72]. *MTHFR C677T* is associated with increased homocysteine levels, a risk factor for vascular events. However, migraine is not associated with elevated levels of homocysteine [73]. Interestingly, coexistence of migraine with aura and the *677TT* genotype selectively raised the risk of ischemic stroke in one cohort study (RR = 4.19; 95%CI = 1.38–12.74) [72], which is support by data from a case-control study [74]. Results of studies evaluating associations between migraine and other genetic polymorphisms that are also associated with vascular risk, such as the *ACE* D/I polymorphism or the beta2 polymorphism, did not find associations with migraine [75,76].

Migraine-specific treatments

Concerns have been raised regarding the cardiovascular safety of the use of migraine medications. Indeed, the use of ergots has been associated with white-matter lesions [14]. However, detailed reviews of the clinical, pharmacological and post-marketing cardiovascular safety data of triptans currently do not support such concerns [77–83]. It is important to note that most of the data from clinical trials and clinical practice regarding the safety of triptans have been derived from patients without known cardiovascular disease [79]. Contraindications for triptans already include existing coronary artery and cardiovascular disease and uncontrolled hypertension. With regard to an increased risk of ischemic events due to triptan therapy, two large-scale studies were recently performed based on records of a health-care provider in the USA [82], and from the General Practice Research Database in the UK [81]. The US database included 130,411 migraine patients and a similar number of controls. Neither current nor recent triptan use was associated with increased risk of myocardial infarction or stroke. The UK database included 63,575 patients with migraine only and also found no association between triptan use and risk of stroke or myocardial infarction or other vascular events. A large claims-based study from The Netherlands evaluated whether overuse of triptans or ergotamins was associated with increased risk of ischemic vascular events [84]. The results of this study indicate that overuse of triptans, even among patients concomitantly using cardiovascular drugs, did not increase the risk of vascular events. In contrast, overuse of ergotamine was associated with an increased risk of vascular events (RR = 2.55; 95% CI = 1.22–5.36), which was further increased for those patients who concomitantly used cardiovascular drugs. Therapeutic doses of either triptans or ergotamine were not associated with increased risk [84].

Diagnosis

In the setting of an ischemic stroke in a patient with migraine, the diagnostic evaluation does not differ from that in a patient without migraine. The most problematic differential diagnosis is the distinction between migraine aura and transient ischemic attacks, at least when migraine aura occurs for the first time or the typical migraine headache is not following the aura. In such circumstances, appropriate brain scans are indicated. In atypical cases of migraine with multiple ischemic strokes (e.g. CADASIL) or with other existing comorbidities, the diagnostic procedures should be extended [3] (see Chapter 3).

Management

Because the absolute risk of stroke is low in young migraine patients, the vast majority of migraine patients will not experience a stroke event. Traditional risk factors for stroke, such as hypertension, smoking, diabetes and obesity, are far more important and should be prevented or treated in young individuals with or without migraine. In addition, since the mechanisms linking migraine with ischemic stroke remain unclear, no overall preventive treatment options can be recommended. Young women with migraine with aura should strongly be advised to stop smoking, and oral contraceptive use should be re-evaluated based on individual risk profiles [85]. Triptans and ergotamine are contraindicated to treat acute migraine attacks in patients with existing cardiovascular disease or uncontrolled hypertension.

There is no direct evidence that treating migraine by any means has an influence on the risk of subsequent vascular events and stroke. Some studies have suggested that low-dose aspirin therapy is associated with a small but significant reduction of migraine frequency [86,87]. Furthermore, it has been shown in a large primary prevention trial that low-dose aspirin reduces the risk of first ischemic stroke in women by 24% [88]. However, this effect was only apparent in women aged 65 years or older, an age group in which migraine prevalence is low. In addition, because of the low absolute risk of stroke in younger age groups but increased risk of major bleeds in all age groups [89], the use of low-dose aspirin for all migraine patients to prevent stroke is not indicated.

It seems particularly important, however, that migraine patients who experience a migraine aura are carefully diagnosed and educated about typical migraine aura features and the difference between these and potential stroke symptoms. This, however, may be difficult when the migraine aura presents with severe focal neurological deficits that even an experienced neurologist cannot distinguish from a stroke symptom. However, in most cases the aura has positive features involving vision, is limited to less than an hour, and is followed by a migraine headache. In the case of a prolonged aura (i.e., a migraine aura symptom >60 minutes) patients should be advised to consult their treating physician. Migraine patients should also consult their physician if their 'typical' aura presents differently. If a migraine patient experiences a stroke, the therapeutic consequences are no different than for any other stroke patient, including detailed work-up, treatment of cardiovascular risk factors, and antiplatelet or anticoagulant therapy to prevent a second stroke. In such patients, ergot derivatives and triptans to treat migraine headache should be avoided.

References

1 Stewart WF, Lipton RB, Celentano DD, Reed ML. Prevalence of migraine headache in the United States: relation to age, income, race, and other sociodemographic factors. JAMA 1992;267:64–9.
2 American Heart Association. Heart Disease and Stroke Statistics. AHA, 2008.
3 Bousser MG, Welch KM. Relation between migraine and stroke. Lancet Neurol 2005;4:533–42.
4 Hargreaves RJ, Shepheard SL. Pathophysiology of migraine – new insights. Can J Neurol Sci 1999;26(Suppl. 3):S12–19.
5 Goadsby PJ. Neurovascular headache and a midbrain vascular malformation: evidence for a role of the brainstem in chronic migraine. Cephalalgia 2002;22:107–11.
6 Henrich JB, Horwitz RI. A controlled study of ischemic stroke risk in migraine patients. J Clin Epidemiol 1989;42:773–80.
7 Chang CL, Donaghy M, Poulter N. Migraine and stroke in young women: case–control study. The World Health Organisation Collaborative Study of Cardiovascular Disease and Steroid Hormone Contraception. Brit Med J 1999;318:13–18.
8 Tzourio C, Bousser MG. Migraine: a risk factor for ischemic stroke in young women. Stroke 1997;28:2569–70.
9 Buring JE, Hebert P, Romero J, et al. Migraine and subsequent risk of stroke in the Physicians' Health Study. Arch Neurol 1995;52:129–34.
10 Kurth T, Slomke MA, Kase CS, et al. Migraine, headache, and the risk of stroke in women: a prospective study. Neurology 2005;64:1020–6.
11 Stang PE, Carson AP, Rose KM, et al. Headache, cerebrovascular symptoms, and stroke: the Atherosclerosis Risk in Communities Study. Neurology 2005;64:1573–7.
12 Etminan M, Takkouche B, Isorna FC, Samii A. Risk of ischaemic stroke in people with migraine: systematic review and meta-analysis of observational studies. Brit Med J 2005;330:63–5.

13 Ziegler DK, Batnitzky S, Barter R, McMillan JH. Magnetic resonance image abnormality in migraine with aura. Cephalalgia 1991;11:147–50.

14 Kruit MC, van Buchem MA, Hofman PA, et al. Migraine as a risk factor for subclinical brain lesions. JAMA 2004;291:427–34.

15 Tzourio C, Tehindrazanarivelo A, Iglesias S, et al. Case-control study of migraine and risk of ischaemic stroke in young women. Brit Med J 1995;310:830–3.

16 Tzourio C, Iglesias S, Hubert JB, et al. Migraine and risk of ischaemic stroke: a case-control study. Brit Med J 1993;307:289–92.

17 Carolei A, Marini C, De Matteis G. History of migraine and risk of cerebral ischaemia in young adults. The Italian National Research Council Study Group on Stroke in the Young. Lancet 1996;347:1503–6.

18 Lidegaard O. Oral contraceptives, pregnancy and the risk of cerebral thromboembolism: the influence of diabetes, hypertension, migraine and previous thrombotic disease. Br J Obstet Gynaecol 1995;102:153–9.

19 Mosek A, Marom R, Korczyn AD, Bornstein N. A history of migraine is not a risk factor to develop an ischemic stroke in the elderly. Headache 2001;41:399–401.

20 Donaghy M, Chang CL, Poulter N. Duration, frequency, recency, and type of migraine and the risk of ischaemic stroke in women of childbearing age. J Neurol Neurosurg Psychiatry. 2002;73:747–50.

21 Schwaag S, Nabavi DG, Frese A, Husstedt IW, Evers S. The association between migraine and juvenile stroke: a case-control study. Headache 2003;43:90–5.

22 Merikangas KR, Fenton BT, Cheng SH, Stolar MJ, Risch N. Association between migraine and stroke in a large-scale epidemiological study of the United States. Arch Neurol 1997;54:362–8.

23 Sochurkova D, Moreau T, Lemesle M, Menassa M, Giroud M, Dumas R. Migraine history and migraine-induced stroke in the Dijon stroke registry. Neuroepidemiology 1999;18:85–91.

24 Milhaud D, Bogousslavsky J, van Melle G, Liot P. Ischemic stroke and active migraine. Neurology 2001;57:1805–11.

25 Collaborative Group for the Study of Stroke in Young Women. Oral contraceptives and stroke in young women: associated risk factors. JAMA 1975;231:718–22.

26 MacClellan LR, Giles WH, Cole J, et al. Probable migraine with visual aura and risk of ischemic stroke: The Stroke Prevention in Young Women Study. Stroke 2007;38:2438–45.

27 Kurth T, Schurks M, Logroscino G, Buring JE. Migraine frequency and risk of cardiovascular disease in women. Neurology 2009;73:581–8.

28 Diener HC, Kurth T. Is migraine a risk factor for stroke? Neurology 2005;64:1496–7.

29 Bushnell CD, Jamison M, James AH. Migraine during pregancies linked to stroke and vascular disease: United States population-based study. Brit Med J 2009;338:6664.

30 Headache Classification Committee of the International Headache Society. The International Classification of Headache Disorders: 2nd edition. Cephalalgia 2004;24(Suppl. 1):9–160.

31 Henrich JB, Sandercock PA, Warlow CP, Jones LN. Stroke and migraine in the Oxfordshire Community Stroke Project. J Neurol 1986;233:257–62.

32 Arboix A, Massons J, Garcia-Eroles L, Oliveres M, Balcells M, Targa C. Migrainous cerebral infarction in the Sagrat Cor Hospital of Barcelona stroke registry. Cephalalgia 2003;23:389–94.

33 Kittner SJ, Stern BJ, Wozniak M, et al. Cerebral infarction in young adults: the Baltimore-Washington Cooperative Young Stroke Study. Neurology 1998;50:890–4.

34 Sacquegna T, Andreoli A, Baldrati A, et al. Ischemic stroke in young adults: the relevance of migrainous infarction. Cephalalgia 1989;9:255–8.

35 D'Anglejan-Chatillon J, Ribeiro V, Mas JL, Youl BD, Bousser MG. Migraine – a risk factor for dissection of cervical arteries. Headache 1989;29:560–1.

36 Tzourio C, Benslamia L, Guillon B, et al. Migraine and the risk of cervical artery dissection: a case-control study. Neurology 2002;59:435–7.

37 Pezzini A, Granella F, Grassi M, et al. History of migraine and the risk of spontaneous cervical artery dissection. Cephalalgia 2005;25:575–80.

38 Silberstein SD, de Lignieres B. Migraine, menopause and hormonal replacement therapy. Cephalalgia 2000;20:214–21.

39 Bushnell CD. Oestrogen and stroke in women: assessment of risk. Lancet Neurol 2005;4:743–51.

40 Vahedi K, Chabriat H, Levy C, Joutel A, Tournier-Lasserve E, Bousser MG. Migraine with aura and brain magnetic resonance imaging abnormalities in patients with CADASIL. Arch Neurol 2004;61:1237–40.

41 Tournier-Lasserve E, Joutel A, Melki J, et al. Cerebral autosomal dominant arteriopathy with subcortical infarcts and leukoencephalopathy maps to chromosome 19q12. Nat Genet 1993;3:256–9.

42 Pavlakis SG, Phillips PC, DiMauro S, De Vivo DC, Rowland LP. Mitochondrial myopathy, encephalopathy, lactic acidosis, and strokelike episodes: a distinctive clinical syndrome. Ann Neurol 1984;16:481–8.

43 Terwindt GM, Haan J, Ophoff RA, et al. Clinical and genetic analysis of a large Dutch family with autosomal dominant vascular retinopathy, migraine and Raynaud's phenomenon. Brain 1998;121:303–16.

44 Olesen J, Friberg L, Olsen TS, et al. Ischaemia-induced (symptomatic) migraine attacks may be more frequent than migraine-induced ischaemic insults. Brain 1993;116:187–202.

45 Mitsias P, Ramadan NM. Headache in ischemic cerebrovascular disease. Part I: Clinical features. Cephalalgia 1992;12:269–74.

46 Leira R, Davalos A, Aneiros A, Serena J, Pumar JM, Castillo J. Headache as a surrogate marker of the molecular mechanisms implicated in progressing stroke. Cephalalgia 2002;22:303–8.

47 Tentschert S, Wimmer R, Greisenegger S, Lang W, Lalouschek W. Headache at stroke onset in 2196 patients with ischemic stroke or transient ischemic attack. Stroke 2005;36:e1–3.

48 Hossmann KA. Periinfarct depolarizations. Cerebrovasc Brain Metab Rev 1996;8:195–208.

49 Wiehe M, Fuchs SC, Moreira LB, Moraes RS, Fuchs FD. Migraine is more frequent in individuals with optimal and normal blood pressure: a population-based study. J Hypertens 2002;20:1303–6.

50 Tzourio C, Gagniere B, El Amrani M, Alperovitch A, Bousser MG. Relationship between migraine, blood pressure and carotid thickness. A population-based study in the elderly. Cephalalgia 2003;23:914–20.

51 Cook NR, Bensenor IM, Lotufo PA, et al. Migraine and coronary heart disease in women and men. Headache 2002;42:715–27.

52 Scher AI, Terwindt GM, Picavet HS, Verschuren WM, Ferrari MD, Launer LJ. Cardiovascular risk factors and migraine: the GEM population-based study. Neurology 2005;64:614–20.

53 Wilson PWF, D'Agostino RB, Levy D, Belanger AM, Silbershatz H, Kannel WB. Prediction of coronary heart disease using risk factor categories. Circulation 1998;97:1837–47.

54 Bigal ME, Liberman JN, Lipton RB. Obesity and migraine: a population study. Neurology 2006;66:545–50.

55 Winter AC, Berger K, Buring JE, Kurth T. Body mass index, migraine, migraine frequency and migraine features in women. Cephalalgia 2009;29:269–78.

56 Kurth T, Gaziano JM, Cook NR, Logroscino G, Diener HC, Buring JE. Migraine and risk of cardiovascular disease in women. JAMA 2006;296:283–91.

57 Kurth T, Gaziano JM, Cook N, et al. Migraine and risk of cardiovascular disease in men. Arch Intern Med 2007;167:795–801.

58 Liew G, Wang JJ, Mitchell P. Migraine and coronary heart disease mortality: a prospective cohort study. Cephalalgia 2007;27:368–71.

59 Kurth T, Schurks M, Logroscino G, Gaziano JM, Buring JE. Migraine, vascular risk, and cardiovascular events in women: prospective cohort study. Brit Med J 2008;337:a636.

60 Anzola GP, Magoni M, Guindani M, Rozzini L, Dalla Volta G. Potential source of cerebral embolism in migraine with aura: a transcranial Doppler study. Neurology 1999;52:1622–5.

61 Schwerzmann M, Nedeltchev K, Lagger F, et al. Prevalence and size of directly detected patent foramen ovale in migraine with aura. Neurology 2005;65:1415–18.

62 Diener HC, Kurth T, Dodick D. Patent foramen ovale, stroke, and cardiovascular disease in migraine. Curr Opin Neurol 2007;20:310–19.

63 Bousser MG. Patent foramen ovale and migraine: evidence for a link? Headache Currents 2006;3:44–51.

64 Rodes-Cabau J, Mineau S, Marrero A, et al. Incidence, timing, and predictive factors of new-onset migraine headache attack after transcatheter closure of atrial septal defect or patent foramen ovale. Am J Cardiol 2008;101:688–92.

65 Schwedt TJ, Demaerschalk BM, Dodick DW. Patent foramen ovale and migraine: a quantitative systematic review. Cephalalgia 2008;28:531–40.

66 Rundek T, Elkind MS, Di Tullio MR, et al. Patent foramen ovale and migraine: a cross-sectional study from the Northern Manhattan Study (NOMAS). Circulation 2008;118:1419–24.

67 Ophoff RA, Terwindt GM, Vergouwe MN, et al. Familial hemiplegic migraine and episodic ataxia type-2 are caused by mutations in the Ca^{2+} channel gene CACNL1A4. Cell 1996;87:543–52.

68 Kors EE, van den Maagdenberg AM, Plomp JJ, Frants RR, Ferrari MD. Calcium channel mutations and migraine. Curr Opin Neurol 2002;15:311–16.

69 De Fusco M, Marconi R, Silvestri L, et al. Haploinsufficiency of ATP1A2 encoding the Na^+/K^+ pump alpha2 subunit associated with familial hemiplegic migraine type 2. Nat Genet 2003;33:192–6.

70 Lea RA, Ovcaric M, Sundholm J, Solyom L, Macmillan J, Griffiths LR. Genetic variants of angiotensin converting enzyme and methylenetetrahydrofolate reductase may act in combination to increase migraine susceptibility. Brain Res Mol Brain Res 2005;136:112–17.

71 Scher AI, Terwindt GM, Verschuren WM, et al. Migraine and MTHFR C677T genotype in a population-based sample. Ann Neurol 2006;59:372–5.

72 Schurks M, Zee RY, Buring JE, Kurth T. Interrelationships among the MTHFR 677C>T polymorphism, migraine, and cardiovascular disease. Neurology 2008;71:505–13.

73 Kurth T, Ridker PM, Buring JE. Migraine and biomarkers of cardiovascular disease in women. Cephalalgia 2008;28:49–56.

74 Pezzini A, Grassi M, Del Zotto E, et al. Migraine mediates the influence of C677T MTHFR genotypes on ischemic stroke risk with a stroke-subtype effect. Stroke 2007;38:3145–51.

75 Schurks M, Kurth T, Ridker PM, Buring JE, Zee RY. Association between polymorphisms in the beta2-adrenoceptor gene and migraine in women. Headache 2009;49:235–44.

76 Schurks M, Zee RY, Buring JE, Kurth T. ACE D/I polymorphism, migraine, and cardiovascular disease in women. Neurology 2009;72:650–6.

77 Welch KM, Mathew NT, Stone P, Rosamond W, Saiers J, Gutterman D. Tolerability of sumatriptan: clinical trials and post-marketing experience. Cephalalgia 2000;20:687–95.

78 Mathew NT, Hettiarachchi J, Alderman J. Tolerability and safety of eletriptan in the treatment of migraine: a comprehensive review. Headache 2003;43:962–74.

79 Dodick DW, Martin VT, Smith T, Silberstein S. Cardiovascular tolerability and safety of triptans: a review of clinical data. Headache 2004;44:S20–30.

80 Maassen Van Den Brink A, Saxena PR. Coronary vasoconstrictor potential of triptans: a review of in vitro pharmacologic data. Headache 2004;44(Suppl 1):S13–9.

81 Hall GC, Brown MM, Mo J, MacRae KD. Triptans in migraine: the risks of stroke, cardiovascular disease, and death in practice. Neurology 2004;62:563–8.

82 Velentgas P, Cole JA, Mo J, Sikes CR, Walker AM. Severe vascular events in migraine patients. Headache 2004;44:642–51.

83 Martin VT, Goldstein JA. Evaluating the safety and tolerability profile of acute treatments for migraine. Am J Med 2005;118(Suppl. 1):S36–44.

84 Wammes-van der Heijden EA, Rahimtoola H, Leufkens HG, Tijssen CC, Egberts AC. Risk of ischemic complications related to the intensity of triptan and ergotamine use. Neurology 2006;67:1128–34.

85 Bousser MG, Conard J, Kittner S, et al. Recommendations on the risk of ischaemic stroke associated with use of combined oral contraceptives and hormone replacement therapy in women with migraine. The International Headache Society Task Force on Combined Oral Contraceptives & Hormone Replacement Therapy. Cephalalgia 2000;20:155–6.

86 Buring JE, Peto R, Hennekens CH. Low-dose aspirin for migraine prophylaxis. JAMA 1990;264:1711–13.

87 Diener HC, Hartung E, Chrubasik J, et al. A comparative study of oral acetylsalicylic acid and metoprolol for the prophylactic treatment of migraine. A randomized, controlled, double-blind, parallel group phase III study. Cephalalgia 2001;21:120–8.

88 Ridker PM, Cook NR, Lee IM, et al. A randomized trial of low-dose aspirin in the primary prevention of cardiovascular disease in women. N Engl J Med 2005;352:1293–304.

89 Berger JS, Roncaglioni MC, Avanzini F, Pangrazzi I, Tognoni G, Brown DL. Aspirin for the primary prevention of cardiovascular events in women and men: a sex-specific meta-analysis of randomized controlled trials. JAMA 2006;295:306–13.

3 Cardiovascular Disorders

Ann I. Scher[1] and David W. Dodick[2]

[1] Department of Preventive Medicine and Biometrics, Uniformed Services University, Bethesda, MD, USA

[2] Department of Neurology, Mayo Clinic Arizona, Phoenix, AZ, USA

Introduction

As reviewed in the previous chapter, migraineurs, particularly those with aura, are at increased risk of clinical and subclinical ischemic stroke and white matter lesions [1–3]. While evidence initially suggested the excess risk of ischemic stroke in migraineurs to be most evident in younger (<45 years) women with aura [3], increased risk has also been described in men and in middle-aged or older male and female migraineurs [4–9].

The mechanism(s) relating migraine with aura and ischemic stroke are likely complex and bidirectional, and may involve both atherosclerotic and non-atherosclerotic pathways as well as methodological artifact [3]. For example, in population and even clinical studies, a small amount of misclassification (e.g. of the migraine aura and transient ischemic attack) may spuriously increase the risk of stroke associated with migraine [3,10,11]. However, methodological artifact is less likely to play a role in the relationship between migraine with aura and other forms of cardiovascular disease (CVD). Other mechanisms to consider that may explain the relationship between migraine and CVD include vasoconstrictor medications taken to treat migraine, classic cardiovascular risk factors, and shared genetic risk factors.

As migraine with aura appears to be a marker or risk factor for ischemic stroke, it is of interest whether there is a similar relationship between migraine with aura and other forms of cardiovascular disease. In this chapter, we review the epidemiologic evidence related to risk of (non-stroke) CVD events associated with migraine, and cardiovascular risk profiles of migraine sufferers.

Epidemiology of migraine and cardiovascular disease

In Table 3.1, the epidemiologic evidence relating to migraine and cardiovascular outcomes other than stroke is summarized. Studies were included if they were based on non-clinical or population-based samples.

Comorbidity in Migraine, First Edition. Edited by J. Schoenen, D. W. Dodick and P. S. Sándor.
© 2011 Blackwell Publishing Ltd. Published 2011 by Blackwell Publishing Ltd.

Table 3.1 Risk of non-stroke cardiovascular disease from non-clinical populations.

Mig or MA	Author	Source	Study subjects	Age	Risk or odds of CHD in migraineurs vs non-migraineurs [95% CI]	CHD outcome
Prospective cohort studies						
MA	Gudmundsson et al. 2010 [8]	Reykjavik Cohort	18,725	33–81	1.28 [1.1–1.5]	CHD Mortality
MA[*]	Kurth et al. 2006 [7][†]	Women's Health Study	27,840 women	45+	1.7 [1.2–2.5] 2.1 [1.3–3.3] 1.7 [1.2–2.5]	Coronary revascularization Myocardial infarction Angina
Mig[‡]	Kurth et al. 2007 [4]	Physicians' Health Study	20,084 men	40+	1.1 [0.9–1.2] 1.4 [1.2–1.8] 1.2 [1.0–1.3]	Coronary revascularization Myocardial infarction Angina
MA[§]	Liew et al. 2007 [15]	Blue Mountain Eye Study	2331	49+	2.2 [0.8–5.8] (♀) No CHD deaths (♂)	CHD death
MA[**]	Rose et al. 2004 [13]	ARIC – community	12,409	45–64	0.7–1.1, all NS 3.0 [2.4–3.7] (♀) 2.2 [1.2–3.9] (♂)	Fatal/non-fatal CHD Rose angina
Mig[††]	Sternfeld et al. 1995 [14]	Kaiser Permanente	79,588	Adults	0.6–1.5, all NS	Fatal/non-fatal MI
Cross-sectional studies						
Mig[‡‡]	Cook NR et al. 1989 [23]	Community	3811	65+	1.4, $p < 0.002$ 1.7, $p < 0.001$	Self-reported history of MI Self-reported history of angina
Mig[§§]	Mitchell et al. 1998 [30]	Blue Mountain Eye Study	3654	49+	1.8 [1.3–2.5] 1.5 [1.2–2.1]	Self-reported history of MI Self-reported history of angina
Mig[***]	Abramson et al. 1982 [20]	Community	3808	25–69	3.6 [1.9–6.8] 1.7 [NS]	Congestive cardiac failure CHD (electrocardiographic evidence)

[*] Aura definition: had an 'aura or any indication a migraine is coming'.
[†] Reanalysis with additional follow-up of study by Cook et al., in which no relationship was seen between migraine and CHD for men or women.
[‡] Self-reported migraine.
[§] IHS diagnostic criteria for migraine with or without aura.
[**] Headaches lasting 4+ hours, modified IHS criteria; aura refers to visual aura.
[††] Pre-IHS criteria or self-reported migraine.
[‡‡] Two of three symptoms: unilateral, nausea, aura ('warning a headache is coming').
[§§] Modified IHS criteria.
[***] Recurrent headache with two or more of visual aura, unilateral location, nausea or vomiting.
CVD, cardiovascular disease; CHD, coronary heart disease; IHS, international headache society; MA, migraine with aura; MI, myocardial infarction; Mig, migraine; NS, not statistically significant.
Data preferentially shown for migraine with aura (MA) when provided.

Case definitions for migraine are shown for each study, and results are shown preferentially for migraine with aura if possible. Studies are further divided into prospective studies (e.g., migraineurs and non-migraineurs are identified and then followed for incident CVD outcomes) and cross-sectional or case-control studies (e.g. migraineurs and non-migraineurs and identified at the same time that CVD outcomes are assessed). Almost all of the studies used non-standardized diagnostic criteria for migraine, and few studies provide results separately for migraine with aura. Nonetheless, some general patterns can be observed within the methodological limitations of the studies to date.

Women's Health Study and Physicians' Health Study

A secondary analysis of the landmark longitudinal Women's Health Study and Physicians' Health Study was conducted in order to consider whether migraine predicted incident ischemic vascular disease, including stroke, myocardial infarction (MI), angina and coronary revascularization. Both studies were clinical trials, had similar methodology, and were initially negative in the first analysis (published in 2002) [12] and positive in the second analysis with additional follow-up (published in 2006/2007) [4,7].

The Physicians' Health Study was a randomized controlled trial of aspirin and beta-carotene to prevent cardiovascular disease and cancer. Study subjects were male physicians age 40+ at baseline, initially free of cardiovascular disease or cancer, who were followed for 13 years (in the 2002 analysis) [12] and for 16 years (in the 2007 analysis) [4]. The incidence of various outcomes (ischemic stroke, MI, coronary revascularization, angina and cardiovascular death) was compared between the men with and without self-reported migraine. This study did not assess the presence of aura. Results from the 2002 analysis were negative, with no difference in risk of the measured outcomes between the men with and without self-reported migraine. However, with additional follow-up, self-reported migraineurs were found to be at increased risk for major cardiovascular events [hazard ratio (HR) = 1.24; 95% confidence interval (CI) = 1.1–1.5], primarily driven by myocardial infarction (HR = 1.4; 95% CI = 1.2–1.8). Migraineurs were not found to be at increased risk of coronary revascularization, angina or cardiovascular death.

The Women's Health Study was a randomized controlled trial of aspirin and vitamin E in the primary prevention of cardiovascular disease or cancer. Participants were female health professionals age 45+ at baseline, initially free of cardiovascular disease or cancer, who were followed for 6 years (2002 analysis) [12] and for 10 years (2006 analysis) [7]. The incidence of various outcomes (ischemic stroke, MI, coronary revascularization, angina and cardiovascular death) was compared between the women with and without self-reported migraine. Aura was positive if the women indicated they had an 'aura or any indication a migraine was coming'. Results from the 2002 analysis were negative, with no difference in risk of the CV-related outcomes between the women with and without migraine. However, with additional follow-up, increased risk was found for the women with active self-reported aura for all cardiovascular events including myocardial infarction (HR = 2.1; 95% CI = 1.3–3.3), coronary revascularization (HR = 1.7; 95% CI = 1.2–2.5) and angina (HR = 1.7; 95% CI = 1.2–2.5). The major limitation of this result is the aura definition, presumably leading to contamination of the aura group with migraineurs who experience non-specific prodromal features. Such misclassification would arguably have attenuated the results if there was a true positive association between migraine with aura and CVD.

A population-based study by Rose et al., the Atherosclerosis Risk In Communities (ARIC) Study, looked at the association between headaches lasting four or more hours, Rose angina, and incident fatal or non-fatal CVD including MI and coronary revascularization procedures [13]. Study participants were aged 45–64 at baseline in 1987, although migraine history was assessed in 1993–95 when the study participants were aged 60 on average. Headache diagnosis was based on a modification of IHS criteria and included an assessment of visual aura ('spots, jagged lines or heat waves in one or both eyes'). Compared to those without a history of headaches lasting four or more hours, the headache group was roughly twice as likely to have a history of Rose angina at baseline, with the risk most elevated in the headache group with aura. Nonetheless, there was no increased risk of incident CVD in any headache group, although the men with non-migraine headaches without aura had a modestly *decreased* risk of incident CVD. Results are consistent with an earlier study by Sternfeld et al. based on a large managed care cohort [14]. In that study, which used non-standardized migraine diagnoses and did not assess aura, migraineurs were also more likely to report chest pain at baseline but were not at increased risk of subsequent MI, with the exception of female migraineurs with a family history of MI.

Liew et al. [15] reported on an Australian population-based cohort of older (49+) men and women. Study subjects were diagnosed with migraine with and without aura using IHS criteria in face-to-face interviews and were followed for six years. Results indicated that women with migraine with aura were at roughly doubled risk of incident CVD death compared to women without migraine [relative risk (RR) = 2.2; 95% CI = 0.8–5.8], although results did not reach statistical significance. There were no CVD-related deaths in the male migraineurs. Results from three cross-sectional studies, generally positive, are also shown in Table 3.1.

In a recent meta-analysis of studies that evaluated the association between migraine and CVD, including stroke, MI and death due to CVD, migraine was associated with a two-fold increased risk of ischemic stroke (pooled RR = 1.73; 95% CI = 1.31–2.29), which was only apparent among people who have migraine with aura (2.16; 95% CI = 1.53–3.03) [16]. The association between migraine and MI (1.12; 95%; CI = 0.95–1.32) and migraine and death due to CVD (1.03; 95% CI = 0.79–1.34) was not significant. While individual studies demonstrated a two-fold increased risk of MI, angina and death due to CVD for people who have migraine with aura, the pooled results from this meta-analysis did not suggest an association between migraine overall and MI, or death due to CVD, whereas the risk of angina was increased by 30%.

After this meta-analysis was published, Gudmundsson et al [8] reported on mortality risk by migraine status in a longitudinal population-based study of more than 18,000 adults. Over more than 25 years of follow-up, compared to controls, subjects with MA were at increased risk of incident all-cause mortality (RR = 1.21 [1.12–1.30]), including mortality due to CHD (RR = 1.28 [1.11–1.49]) and stroke (RR = 1.40 [1.10–1.78]).

In summary, the degree to which migraine is related to risk of CVD remains uncertain based on the evidence to date. While it is likely that increased risk, if any, would be most evident for those experiencing aura, the assessment of aura in most of the studies to date is problematic. Further, most studies assessed migraine in middle age or later – leading to the possibility of recall error or selective mortality. Evidence does suggest a more robust relationship between migraine and chest pain or angina, although the mechanism behind this association is uncertain.

Migraine, triptans and cardiovascular disease
Triptans are contraindicated or used with caution in those with pre-existing CVD or those believed to be at risk of CVD:

Risk of Myocardial Ischemia and/or Infarction and Other Adverse Cardiac Events: Sumatriptan should not be given to patients with documented ischemic or vasospastic coronary artery disease (CAD) (see CONTRAINDICATIONS). It is strongly recommended that sumatriptan not be given to patients in whom unrecognized CAD is predicted by the presence of risk factors (e.g., hypertension, hypercholesterolemia, smoker, obesity, diabetes, strong family history of CAD, female with surgical or physiological menopause, or male over 40 years of age) unless a cardiovascular evaluation provides satisfactory clinical evidence that the patient is reasonably free of coronary artery and ischemic myocardial disease or other significant underlying cardiovascular disease. The sensitivity of cardiac diagnostic procedures to detect cardiovascular disease or predisposition to coronary artery vasospasm is modest, at best. If, during the cardiovascular evaluation, the patient's medical history or electrocardiographic investigations reveal findings indicative of, or consistent with, coronary artery vasospasm or myocardial ischemia, sumatriptan should not be administered (see CONTRAINDICATIONS).

For patients with risk factors predictive of CAD, who are determined to have a satisfactory cardiovascular evaluation, it is strongly recommended that administration of the first dose of sumatriptan tablets takes place in the setting of a physician's office or similar medically staffed and equipped facility unless the patient has previously received sumatriptan. Because cardiac ischemia can occur in the absence of clinical symptoms, consideration should be given to obtaining on the first occasion of use an electrocardiogram (ECG) during the interval immediately following IMITREX Tablets, in these patients with risk factors.

"Extracted from sumatriptan prescribing information [17]

In observational studies, therefore, the expectation is that migraineurs who are prescribed triptans would be at reduced risk of CVD compared to migraineurs who are not prescribed triptans. Observational studies that compare cardiovascular outcomes in triptan-using versus non-triptan-using migraineurs are thus inherently confounded by indication in a way that would be expected to attenuate or reverse any theoretical increased risk of cardiovascular disease in migraineurs; adjustment for known risk profiles can only partly control for this inherent limitation.

Such studies can address, however, whether the use of triptans (and ergotamine) *in practice* is associated with risk of cardiovascular outcomes. Two such studies [18,19] based on managed care samples performed this analysis and are summarized below. Migraine sufferers were identified through medical records based on diagnostic history and/or prescription of migraine-specific medication. Various cardiovascular outcomes were assessed through diagnostic codes as detailed below. Data were analyzed to determine whether migraineurs thus identified were at increased risk of incident cardiovascular disease compared to non-migraineurs. Additional analyses were performed to determine the extent to which risk was related to the use of triptans [18,19] or ergotamine [18]. Risk ratios in both studies were adjusted by baseline diagnosed and coded cardiovascular risk factors.

The first study by Velentgas et al. [18] was based on 260,822 members of UnitedHealthcare. Migraineurs were identified based on diagnostic history or history of triptan use. In this study, the baseline risk of diagnosed migraine was not associated with incident MI or serious ventricular arrhythmia. However, migraineurs were more likely to experience unstable angina (RR = 1.33; 95% CI = 1.1–1.6) than controls. In addition, migraineurs at baseline were more likely to have had *past* CVD [odds ratio (OR) =1.7; 95% CI = 1.5–1.9, estimated] . The risk of death was non-significantly lower in the migraineurs compared to the non-migraineurs (RR = 0.92; 95% CI = 0.8–1.1). Among migraineurs, rates of most outcomes were similar between triptan and non-triptan users although unstable angina and all-cause mortality was lower in the current triptan-using migraineurs compared to the non-triptan-using migraineurs. Among migraineurs, use of ergot alkaloid medication was associated with increased risk of all-cause mortality but not cardiovascular related outcomes. It should be noted that triptan users were likely over-represented due to the selection criteria used for this study (38% of migraineurs).

In the second study by Hall et al., diagnosed migraineurs and matched controls were identified from the General Practice Research Database in the UK [19]. Outcomes considered included MI, ischemic heart disease, ventricular arrhythmia, all-cause mortality and cardiovascular mortality. In this cohort, migraine was associated with increased risk of fatal or non-fatal ischemic heart disease (RR = 1.3; 95% CI = 1.2–1.4). While the triptan- and non-triptan-using migraineurs were not compared directly, this increased risk appeared roughly comparable in the two groups. However, migraineurs were at decreased risk of all-cause mortality compared to non-migraineurs (RR = 0.76; 95% CI = 0.7–0.8). The authors noted that triptans were prescribed to those at less risk of these outcomes.

Migraine and cardiovascular risk factors

A number of population studies have presented data related to cardiovascular risk profiles in migraineurs – mostly in the context of studying baseline risk factors when the outcome of interest was stroke or coronary heart disease [7, 12, 13, 14, 20–42]. While not the primary aim of these studies, some studies reported a higher prevalence of some – but not all – markers of cardiovascular risk, with the most consistent findings related to use of oral contraceptives/hormone replacement therapy (HRT) [7, 31, 32, 34, 42], low alcohol intake [7, 12, 26, 29, 34, 36], and, as previously mentioned, chest pain or angina [7, 13, 14, 20, 24, 31].

Two studies [30,34] specifically examined cardiovascular risk profiles in migraine sufferers with and without aura. The first study, from the GEM (Genetic Epidemiology of Migraine) Study, was based on a random sample of men and women aged 20 to 65 from The Netherlands [33]. Migraine with and without aura was diagnosed using standardized criteria, and diagnosis was supervised by expert headache diagnosticians. Study subjects were asked to draw their visual symptoms, if reported. Results from this suggested that the migraineurs, particularly those with aura, were more likely to have a negative cholesterol profile – high total cholesterol or low high-density lipoproteins (HDL) or high total cholesterol/HDL ratio – high blood pressure, parental history of early MI, and other risk factors. Elevated blood pressure was found only in the migraineurs who had not consulted physicians for their headaches. The authors speculated that migraineurs who had consulted physicians may have received headache-specific treatment that lowered their blood pressure or had been diagnosed with high blood pressure. This study also found that the women with migraine were more likely to have been diagnosed with gestational hypertension.

The second study, an analysis from the Women's Health Study [30], specifically measured biomarkers of cardiovascular risk in migraineurs and non-migraineurs. Significant, but mostly modest, increases were found in some biomarkers of cardiovascular risk including total cholesterol, low-density lipoproteins (LDL), HDL and non-HDL cholesterol, apolipoprotein B_{100}, C-reactive protein and soluble intercellular adhesion molecule 1. In contrast to the results from the GEM study, cardiovascular risk profiles did not appear to be related to the presence of aura – although limitations of the aura definition used in this study have been previously noted.

A relatively common variant in the methylenetetrahydrofolate reductase enzyme (MTHFR C677T), a key enzyme in the metabolism of folate, results in moderately increased plasma homocysteine, particularly when dietary intake of folic acid is low [43, 44]. Increased homocysteine and/or the *MTHFR C677T* genotype have been linked to increased risk of stroke and possibly coronary heart disease in observational studies [43, 45, 46], although clinical trials of folic acid for secondary prevention of cardiovascular disease have primarily been negative [47]. Several clinic-based studies [48–52] and one population study [53] have found associations with *MTHFR C677T* homozygosity and migraine – primarily with aura – although other studies have been negative [54,55]. The folate/homocysteine metabolic pathway is thus a plausible mechanistic pathway for the link between migraine with aura and cardiovascular disease. Reasons for the lack of replication in some studies may include publication bias, population genetic variability, or even population differences in folic acid intake. We note that this polymorphism is the only replicated genetic variant found to be associated with a common migraine type; the association between the homocysteine metabolic pathway and migraine is an area of active research.

Pathophysiology

Since the link between migraine and cardiovascular disease has not been established conclusively, the pathophysiological relationship remains uncertain. However, a potential mechanism for such a relationship may be endothelial dysfunction (ED). Endothelial dysfunction and activation are characterized, respectively, by impaired reactivity of the macro and microvasculature and a procoagulant, proinflammatory and proliferative state, which in turn predispose to atherogenesis. Traditional cardiovascular risk factors are known to have significant impact on endothelial dysfunction, and these traditional risk factors appear to be comorbid with migraine. Migraineurs have been shown to have significantly higher levels of glucose and insulin, at fasting and after glucose loading. In one study, after glucose loading, 65% of the migraineurs had an insulin resistance pattern compared to 19% in the control group [56]. The Genetic Epidemiology of Migraine study found that compared to controls, migraineurs are more likely to smoke and are more likely to have a parental history of early MI [34]. The study also found that migraineurs with aura are more likely to have an unfavorable cholesterol profile, elevated blood pressure, report a history of early-onset coronary heart disease or stroke, and have a two-fold increased risk of a high Framingham risk score-predicted 10-year risk of coronary heart disease even after adjusting for age. In another prospective cohort study, the association between migraine with aura and angina was increased for patients in the low and high Framingham risk score groups, but the association between migraine with aura and MI was apparent only among patients with a high Framingham risk score [57]. The authors of this study proposed that the effect of migraine with aura on the coronary arteries might involve two mechanisms, one involving a vasculature not altered by atherosclerosis leading to angina and one involving a vasculature impaired by atherosclerosis leading to angina and MI.

Even in the absence of these traditional risk factors, migraine has been associated with endothelial dysfunction. One of the strongest pieces of evidence demonstrating endothelial dysfunction in migraine sufferers, particularly with aura, is the numerical depletion and increased senescence of endothelial progenitor cells (EPCs) [58]. EPCs replace injured endothelium cells, and therefore prevent the formation of atherosclerotic plaques. The number of circulating EPCs is considered to be a surrogate biological marker of endothelial function and repair capacity, and studies have demonstrated significant reductions in circulating EPCs in patients with ischemic CVD [59]. In a recent study, the mean numbers of EPC colony-forming units were significantly reduced in migraine subjects with aura [58]. In addition, EPCs from migraine patients showed reduced migratory capacity and increased cellular senescence compared with EPCs from controls and individuals with tension-type headache.

These data, among others, suggest that migraine is associated with a systemic endotheliopathy. Individuals with migraine, particularly young patients aged less than 45, have decreased cerebral and peripheral vascular resistance, retinal microvascular signs, and multiple markers of hypercoagulability and inflammation [60–65]. In particular, migraine has been associated with thrombocytosis, polycythemia vera, platelet aggregation, and increased levels of platelet-activating factor, von Willebrand factor (vWF) and tissue plasminogen activator antigen, all of which have been associated with an increased risk of CVD [65]. Ictal studies during migraine attacks have also demonstrated elevated levels of endothelin-1, soluble intercellular adhesion molecule, tissue necrosis factor, transforming growth factor beta 1, and matrix metalloproteinase-9, indicating that the endothelium may be activated directly during a migraine attack [66–69]. In a recent study, women with migraine with aura had higher adjusted odds ratios compared to controls for elevated vWF activity of 6.51 (95% CI = 1.94–21.83), elevated high-sensitivity C-reactive protein of 7.99 (95% CI = 2.32–27.61) and lower nitrate/nitrite levels of 6.60 (95% CI = 2.06–21.16). The authors concluded that in premenopausal women with migraine, particularly in those with migraine with aura, there is evidence of increased endothelial activation, a component of endothelial dysfunction [65].

Diagnosis and management

While definitive evidence linking migraine with ischemic cardiovascular disease is lacking, individuals with migraine should undergo the same vascular assessment as any other patient with independent vascular risk factors, and screened for traditional cardiovascular risk factors, such as hypertension, adverse lipid profile and increased risk of coronary heart disease, and, if appropriate, these risk factors should be modified. This is particularly true for migraineurs with aura, where the risk of ischemic stroke is reasonably well established. This risk is amplified in women younger than 45 years who are concurrent smokers and using oral contraceptives. Thus, in particular, young women who have migraine with aura should be strongly advised to stop smoking, and methods of birth control other than oral contraceptives should be considered.

It is important, however, to bear in mind that the absolute risk of CVD is low in young migraine patients, and that the vast majority of migraine patients will not experience an ischemic stroke or myocardial infarction.

In addition, since the mechanisms linking migraine with ischemic vascular disease remain unclear, no overall preventive treatment options can be recommended. Triptans and ergotamine are contraindicated to treat acute migraine attacks in patients with existing CVD or uncontrolled hypertension. There is no direct evidence that treating migraine with prophylactic therapy has an influence on the risk of subsequent vascular events and stroke. Some studies have suggested that low-dose aspirin therapy is associated with a small but significant reduction of migraine frequency [70,71]. Furthermore, it has been shown in a large primary prevention trial that low-dose aspirin reduces the risk of first ischemic stroke in women by 24% [72]. However, this effect was only apparent in women aged 65 years or older, an age group in which migraine prevalence is low [73]. In addition, because of the low absolute risk of stroke in younger age groups but increased risk of major bleeds in all age groups, the use of low-dose aspirin for all migraine patients to prevent stroke is not indicated.

If a migraine patient experiences a stroke or MI, the diagnostic and therapeutic implications are no different than for any other stroke or MI patient, including detailed cardiac and neurological assessment, treatment of cardiovascular risk factors, and antiplatelet or anticoagulant therapy for secondary prevention. In such patients, ergot derivatives and triptans to treat migraine headache should be avoided.

The ultimate goal should be to elucidate the association, and to target the identification of groups at particular risk of CVD. Until now, most studies focused on migraine as a risk factor for CVD. Future studies should assess the importance of headache frequency and severity, as well as frequency of auras. If headache frequency is a risk factor for CVD, effective prophylactic treatment of migraine may reduce the risk of CVD, and further studies directly evaluating this question are needed.

References

1 Kruit MC, van Buchem MA, Hofman PA, et al. Migraine as a risk factor for subclinical brain lesions. JAMA 2004;291:427–34.

2 Swartz RH, Kern RZ. Migraine is associated with magnetic resonance imaging white matter abnormalities: a meta-analysis. Arch Neurol 2004;61: 1366–8.

3 Bousser MG, Welch KM. Relation between migraine and stroke. Lancet Neurol 2005;Sep 4(9):533–42.

4 Kurth T, Gaziano JM, Cook NR, et al. Migraine and risk of cardiovascular disease in men. Arch Intern Med 2007;167:795–801.

5 Stang PE, Carson AP, Rose KM, et al. Headache, cerebrovascular symptoms, and stroke: the Atherosclerosis Risk in Communities Study. Neurology 2005;64:1573–7.

6 Buring JE, Hebert P, Romero J, et al. Migraine and subsequent risk of stroke in the Physicians' Health Study. Arch Neurol 1995;52:129–34.

7 Kurth T, Gaziano JM, Cook NR, Logroscino G, Diener HC, Buring JE. Migraine and risk of cardiovascular disease in women. JAMA 2006;296:283–91.

8 Gudmundsson LS, Scher AI, Aspelund T et al, Migraine with aura and risk of cardiovascular and all cause mortality in men and women: prospective cohort study, BMJ 2010;341:c3966.

9 Scher AI, Gudmundsson LS, Sigurdsson S, et al, Migraine headache in middle age and late-life brain infarcts, JAMA 2009;301(24):2563–2570.

10 Welch KM. Stroke and migraine – the spectrum of cause and effect. Funct Neurol 2003;18:121–6.

11 Schoenen J, Sándor PS. Headache with focal neurological signs or symptoms: a complicated differential diagnosis. Lancet Neurol 2004; 3:237–45.

12 Cook NR, Bensenor IM, Lotufo PA, et al. Migraine and coronary heart disease in women and men. Headache 2002;42:715–27.

13 Rose KM, Carson AP, Sanford CP, et al. Migraine and other headaches: associations with Rose angina and coronary heart disease. Neurology 2004;63:2233–9.

14 Sternfeld B, Stang P, Sidney S. Relationship of migraine headaches to experience of chest pain and subsequent risk for myocardial infarction. Neurology 1995;45:2135–42.

15 Liew G, Wang JJ, Mitchell P. Migraine and coronary heart disease mortality: a prospective cohort study. Cephalalgia 2007;27:368–371.

16 Schürks M, Rist PM, Bigal ME, et al, Migraine and cardiovascular disease: systematic review and metanalysis, BMJ 2009; 339:b3914.

17 Imitrex (sumatriptan succinate) Prescribing Information. GlaxoSmithKline, 2007.

18 Velentgas P, Cole JA, Mo J, Sikes CR, Walker AM. Severe vascular events in migraine patients. Headache 2004;44:642–51.

19 Hall GC, Brown MM, Mo J, MacRae KD. Triptans in migraine: the risks of stroke, cardiovascular disease, and death in practice. Neurology 2004;62:563–8.

20 Abramson JH, Hopp C, Epstein LM. Migraine and non-migrainous headaches. A community survey in Jerusalem. J Epidemiol Commun H 1980;34:188–93.

21 Abramson JH, Gofin J, Peritz E, Hopp C, Epstein LM. Clustering of chronic disorders – a community study of coprevalence in Jerusalem. J Chronic Dis 1982;35:221–30.

22 Bigal ME, Liberman JN, Lipton RB. Obesity and migraine: A population study. Neurology 2006;66:545–50.

23 Carson AP, Rose KM, Sanford CP, et al. Lifetime prevalence of migraine and other headaches lasting 4 or more hours: the Atherosclerosis Risk in Communities (ARIC) study. Headache 2004;44;20–8.

24 Cook NR, Evans DA, Funkenstein HH, et al. Correlates of headache in a population-based cohort of elderly. Arch Neurol 1989;46:1338–44.

25 D'Alessandro R, Benassi G, Lenzi PL, et al. Epidemiology of headache in the Republic of San Marino. J Neurol Neurosurg Psychiatry 1988;51:21–7.

26 Gilmour H, Wilkins K. Migraine. Health Rep 2001;12:23–40.

27 Gudmundsson LS, Thorgeirsson G, Sigfusson N, Sigvaldason H, Johannsson M. Migraine patients have lower systolic but higher diastolic blood pressure compared with controls in a population-based study of 21 537 subjects. The Reykjavik Study. Cephalalgia 2006;26:436–44.

28 Hagen K, Stovner LJ, Vatten L, Holmen J, Zwart JA, Bovim G. Blood pressure and risk of headache: a prospective study of 22 685 adults in Norway. J Neurol Neurosurg Psychiatry 2002;72:463–6.

29 Jaillard AS, Mazetti P, Kala E. Prevalence of migraine and headache in a high-altitude town of Peru: a population-based study. Headache 1997;37:95–101.

30 Kurth T, Ridker PM, Buring JE. Migraine and biomarkers of cardiovascular disease in women. Cephalalgia 2008;28:49–56.

31 Mitchell P, Wang JJ, Currie J, Cumming RG, Smith W. Prevalence and vascular associations with migraine in older Australians. Aust NZ J Med 1998;28:627–32.

32 Moorhead T, Hannaford P, Warskyj M. Prevalence and characteristics associated with use of hormone replacement therapy in Britain. Br J Obstet Gynaecol 1997;104:290–7.

33 Rasmussen BK. Migraine and tension-type headache in a general population: precipitating factors, female hormones, sleep pattern and relation to lifestyle. Pain 1993;53:65–72.

34 Scher AI, Terwindt GM, Picavet HSJ, Verschuren WMM, Ferrari MD, Launer LJ. Cardiovascular risk factors and migraine: The GEM population-based study. Neurology 2005;64:614–20.

35 Sillanpaa M, Aro H. Headache in teenagers: comorbidity and prognosis. Funct Neurol 2000;15(Suppl. 3):116–21.

36 Takeshima T, Ishizaki K, Fukuhara Y, et al. Population-based door-to-door survey of migraine in Japan: The Daisen Study. Headache 2004;44:8–19.

37 Tzourio C, Gagniere B, El Amrani M, Alperovitch A, Bousser MG. Relationship between migraine, blood pressure and carotid thickness. A population-based study in the elderly. Cephalalgia 2003;23:914–20.

38 Ulrich V, Olesen J, Gervil M, Russell M. Possible risk factors and precipitants for migraine with aura in discordant twin-pairs: a population-based study. Cephalalgia 2000;20:821–5.

39 Wang SJ, Fuh JL, Lu SR, Juang KD, Wang PH. Migraine prevalence during menopausal transition. Headache 2003;43:470–8.

40 Waters WE. Headache and blood pressure in the community. Brit Med J 1971 Jan 16;1(5741):142–3.

41 Wiehe M, Costa FS, Moreira LB, Stoll MR, Fuchs FD. Migraine is more frequent in individuals with optimal and normal blood pressure: a population-based study. J Hypertens 2002;20:1303–6.

42 Aegidius K, Zwart J-A, Hagen K, Schei B, Stovner LJ. Oral contraceptives and increased headache prevalence: The Head-HUNT study. Neurology 2006; 66:349–53.

43 De Bree A, Verschuren WM, Kromhout D, Kluijtmans LA, Blom HJ. Homocysteine determinants and the evidence to what extent homocysteine determines the risk of coronary heart disease. Pharmacol Rev 2002;54: 599–618.

44 de Bree A, Verschuren WM, Bjorke-Monsen AL, et al. Effect of the methylenetetrahydrofolate reductase 677C–>T mutation on the relations among folate intake and plasma folate and homocysteine concentrations in a general population sample. Am J Clin Nutr 2003;77:687–93.

45 Lewis SJ, Ebrahim S, Davey SG. Meta-analysis of MTHFR 677C–>T polymorphism and coronary heart disease: does totality of evidence support causal role for homocysteine and preventive potential of folate? Brit Med J 2005;331:1053.

46 Bautista LE, Arenas IA, Penuela A, Martinez LX. Total plasma homocysteine level and risk of cardiovascular disease: a meta-analysis of prospective cohort studies. J Clin Epidemiol 2002;55:882–7.

47 Bazzano LA, Reynolds K, Holder KN, He J. Effect of folic acid supplementation on risk of cardiovascular diseases: a meta-analysis of randomized controlled trials. JAMA 2006;296:2720–6.

48 Kowa H, Yasui K, Takeshima T, Urakami K, Sakai F, Nakashima K. The homozygous C677T mutation in the methylenetetrahydrofolate reductase gene is a genetic risk factor for migraine. Am J Med Genet 2000;96:762–4.

49 Oterino A, Valle N, Bravo Y, et al. MTHFR T677 homozygosis influences the presence of aura in migraineurs. Cephalalgia 2004;24:491–4.

50 Lea RA, Ovcaric M, Sundholm J, MacMillan J, Griffiths LR. The methylenetetrahydrofolate reductase gene variant C677T influences susceptibility to migraine with aura. BMC Med 2004;2:3.

51 Kara I, Sazci A, Kaya G, Ergul E, Kilic G. Association of the C677T and A1298C polymorphisms in the MTHFR gene with migraine risk. Am J Hum Genet 2002;71:1026.

52 de Tommaso TM, Difruscolo O, Sardaro M, et al. Influence of MTHFR genotype on contingent negative variation and MRI abnormalities in migraine. Headache 2007;47:253–65.

53 Scher AI, Terwindt GM, Verschuren WM, et al. Migraine, MTHFR C677T genotype in a population-based sample. Ann Neurol 2006 Feb;59(2).

54 Todt U, Freudenberg J, Goebel I, et al. MTHFR C677T polymorphism and migraine with aura. Ann Neurol 2006 Nov;60(5):621–2.

55 Kaunisto M, Kallela M, Hamalainen E, et al. Testing of variants of the MTHFR and ESR1 genes in 1798 Finnish individuals fails to confirm the association with migraine with aura. Cephalalgia 2006;26:1462–72.

56 Cavestro C, Rosatello A, Micca G, et al. Insulin metabolism is altered in migraineurs: a new pathogenic mechanism for migraine? Headache 2007;47:1436–42.

57 Kurth T, Schürks M, Logroscino G, Gaziano JM, Buring JE. Migraine. vascular risk, and cardiovascular disease in women. Prospective cohort study. Brit Med J 2008;337;a636; doi:10.1136/bmj.a636.

58 Lee ST, Chu K, Jung KH, et al. Decreased number and function of endothelial progenitor cells in patients with migraine. Neurology 2008;70:1510–17.

59 Kunz GA, Liang G, Cuculi F, et al. Circulating endothelial progenitor cells predict coronary artery disease severity. Am Heart J 2006;152:190–5.

60 Vanmolkot FH, Van Bortel LM, de Hoon JN. Altered arterial function in migraine of recent onset. Neurology 2007;68:1563–70.

61 Rose KM, Wong TY, Carson AP, Couper DJ, Klein R, Sharrett AR. Migraine and retinal microvascular abnormalities: the Atherosclerosis Risk in Communities Study. Neurology 2007;68:1694–700.

62 Totaro R, Marini C, De Matteis G, Di Napoli M, Carolei A. Cerebrovascular reactivity in migraine during headache-free intervals. Cephalalgia 1997;17:191–4.

63 Tietjen GE, Al-Qasmi MM, Athanas K, Utley C, Herial NA. Altered hemostasis in migraineurs studied with a dynamic flow system.Thromb Res 2007;119:217–222.

64 Longoni M, Ferrarese C. Inflammation and excitotoxicity: role in migraine pathogenesis. Neurol Sci 2006;27(Suppl. 2):S107–10.

65 Tietjen GE, Herial NA, White L, Utley C, Kosmyna JM, Khuder SA. Migraine and biomarkers of endothelial activation in young women. Stroke 2009;40:2977–82.

66 Gallai V, Sarchielli P, Firenze C, et al. Endothelin-1 in migraine and tension-type headache. Acta Neurol Scand 1994;89:47–55.

67 Sarchielli P, Alberti A, Baldi A, et al. Proinflammatory cytokines, adhesion molecules, and lymphocyte integrin expression in the internal jugular blood of migraine patients without aura assessed ictally. Headache 2006;46:200–7.

68 Ishizaki K, Takeshima T, Fukuhara Y, et al. Increased plasma transforming growth factor-1 in migraine. Headache 2005;45:1224 –8.

69 Leira R, Sobrino T, Rodriguez-Yanez M, Blanco M, Arias S, Castillo J. MMP-9 immunoreactivity in acute migraine. Headache 2007;47:698–702.

70 Buring JE, Peto R, Hennekens CH. Low-dose aspirin for migraine prophylaxis. JAMA 1990;264:1711–13.

71 Diener HC, Hartung E, Chrubasik J, et al. A comparative study of oral acetylsalicylic acid and metoprolol for the prophylactic treatment of migraine. A randomized, controlled, double-blind, parallel group phase III study. Cephalalgia 2001;21:120–8.

72 Ridker PM, Cook NR, Lee IM, et al. A randomized trial of low-dose aspirin in the primary prevention of cardiovascular disease in women. N Engl J Med. 2005;352:1293–304.

73 Berger JS, Roncaglioni MC, Avanzini F, Pangrazzi I, Tognoni G, Brown DL. Aspirin for the primary prevention of cardiovascular events in women and men: a sex-specific meta-analysis of randomized controlled trials. JAMA 2006;295:306–13.

4 Patent Foramen Ovale and Migraine

Todd J. Schwedt[1] and Jean Schoenen[2]

[1] Washington University Headache Center, Washington University School of Medicine, St Louis, MO, USA
[2] Headache Research Unit, Department of Neurology & GIGA-Neurosciences, Liège University, Liège, Belgium

Case report

A 34-year-old woman presents to your office with a chief complaint of headaches. She reports having headaches since 14 years of age, with onset shortly after menarche. Initially she had headaches 1–2 days per month, but frequency has increased gradually over the years to the current pattern of 12 severe headache days and 10 mild headache days per month. Severe headaches are unilateral, throbbing, associated with photophobia, phonophobia, nausea and vomiting. She feels disabled and requires bed rest on many of her severe headache days. Approximately 80% of her severe headaches are preceded by visual and sensory phenomena. She describes scintillating scotoma and paresthesias of the fingers and arm on the side ipsilateral to the headache. These symptoms progress slowly over 10–15 minutes and resolve completely within 30 minutes of when headache pain begins.

The patient currently treats with her allotted nine pills of a triptan for severe headaches each month and does not use abortive therapy for milder headaches in order to avoid medication overuse headache. The triptan usually lessens her pain level, although it does not completely abort the pain. She has tried multiple other abortives without greater success. Current prophylactics include topiramate 100 mg q.h.s. and amitriptyline 100 mg q.h.s. She has had adequate trials with several antiepileptics, antidepressants, blood pressure medications, vitamins, supplements and complementary therapy. She has never had great success with any of these prophylactic regimens.

She has no significant past medical history and does not take any other medications. Her mother and sister have both been diagnosed with migraine with aura.

Her vital signs, physical and neurologic examinations are normal.

The patient had a recent magnetic resonance imaging (MRI) scan of the brain, with and without gadolinium, ordered by her primary care physician. MRI showed several punctuate hyperintensities on T2-weighted images in the subcortical white matter of the right and left frontal lobes. These did not

Comorbidity in Migraine, First Edition. Edited by J. Schoenen, D. W. Dodick and P. S. Sándor.
© 2011 Blackwell Publishing Ltd. Published 2011 by Blackwell Publishing Ltd.

display gadolinium enhancement, and diffusion-weighted images were normal. The rest of the MRI was normal.

Her primary care physician, recently having heard news reports on the association between patent foramen ovale (PFO) and migraine, ordered a transthoracic echocardiogram with peripheral injection of agitated saline. This study showed normal cardiac function and size but was positive for right-to-left shunt suggestive of a moderately sized PFO.

The primary care physician suggested that the patient see a headache specialist for discussion of PFO closure. The patient is in your office asking for your opinion. She is hopeful that PFO closure will finally provide her with migraine relief and is willing to undergo the procedure.

Introduction

An increased prevalence of patent foramen ovale (PFO) has been found in patients who have migraine with aura (MA). An increased prevalence of MA is found in patients with PFO. Despite recognition of this association between PFO and MA, the nature of the relationship between these two entities is unclear. It is possible that the two conditions occur coincidentally, or are coinherited, or there may be a causal or triggering relationship with PFO predisposing to MA episodes. The possibility of a causal relationship has led to prospective, randomized, sham-controlled trials of PFO closure for the prophylaxis against migraine. In this chapter, we discuss data supporting an association between PFO and migraine, anatomy of a PFO, hypotheses as to the nature of the association between PFO and migraine, review data regarding PFO closure for migraine, and discuss areas for additional investigation.

Anatomy of a PFO

A PFO is a tunnel-like opening that connects the right and left atria of the heart. The foramen ovale is a necessary component of fetal circulation allowing oxygenated blood to flow from the right atrium to the left atrium. After birth when left atrial pressures exceed those in the right atrium, the septum primum and septum secundum usually join and fuse. If they do not contact one another, the result is an atrial septal defect. If they make contact but the flap-like covering in the left atrium does not fuse, the result is a PFO. During conditions when right atrial pressures are great enough to cause opening of this non-fused flap-like valve, right-to-left shunting occurs. In a patient with an otherwise normal heart, this may occur during each cardiac cycle, with maneuvers further increasing pressures such as Valsalva, and in patients with flow from the inferior vena cava directed towards the PFO [1,2].

Right-to-left shunt results in bypass of the pulmonary circulation, which usually acts as an important filter of particulate matter and metabolites of venous blood. The pulmonary capillaries can trap small emboli prior to entry into the arterial circulation. Right-to-left shunt may thus allow these emboli, which would normally be filtered in the lungs, to reach the brain and other organs. In addition, the lungs play an important role in the

(a)

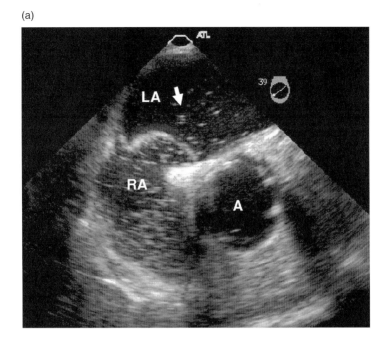

(b)   cTCD in a chronic migraine patient with PFO

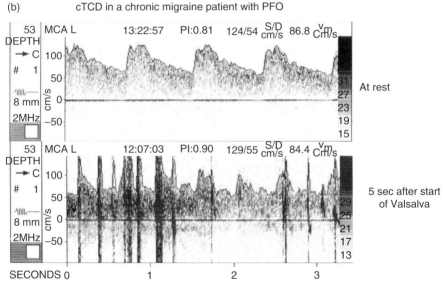

Figure 4.1 (a) Contrast transesophageal echocardiography showing penetration of multiple microbubbles (arrow) from right atrium (RA) into left atrium (LA) through a patent foramen ovale. Note that the PFO is accompanied in this case by an aneurysm of the atrial septum. A, aorta. Reproduced from Schoenen et al. [7] with permission from Revue Médicale de Liège.
(b) Transcranial Doppler in a chronic migraine patient: upper recording at rest during normal breathing; lower recording starting 5 s after a Valsalva maneuver that began 5 s after the contrast injection and showing multiple 'blots', some grouped in a 'curtain'. Multidop DWI, 2-MHz pulsed probe, left middle cerebral artery insonated over a temporal window at a 53 mm depth, contrast medium 9 mL saline + 1 mL air flushed 10 times before injection.

removal of biogenic amines such as norepinephrine (noradrenaline) and
serotonin. Serotonin is extensively extracted and then degraded by
monoamine oxidase during a single pass through the pulmonary circulation.
It is estimated that 80–95% of serotonin is cleared by the lungs [3].
Paradoxical emboli and increased concentrations of vasoactive substances
reaching the arterial system via bypass of the lungs have been proposed as
mechanisms for PFO-related diseases. Larger PFOs with more active shunts
are thus thought to be more likely associated with disease states.

The diagnosis of PFO may be made by transthoracic echocardiography
(cTTE), transesophageal echocardiography (cTEE) or transcranial Doppler
ultrasound (cTCD) (Figure 4.1) with peripheral injection of agitated
contrast. All of these modalities depend upon injection of agitated contrast
into a peripheral vein and imaging for appearance of bubbles either in the
left atrium or in the middle cerebral artery. This is performed with the
patient at rest and with Valsalva maneuver. The degree of right-to-left
shunting is determined by counting the number of bubbles appearing
within a predetermined time period, often three to five cardiac cycles. Two
grading scales are in use. The International Consensus Classification (ICC)
[3] comprises three grades: grade 1, <10 microbubbles; grade 2, ≥10; grade
3, a curtain of bubbles. Spencer's Logarithmic Scale [4] has five grades: 1:
0–10; 2: 11–30; 3: 31–100; 4: 101–300; 5: >300. The ICC grade 3 and
Spencer grades ≥3 correspond to large shunts with a high sensitivity and
specificity [5]. cTEE (Figure 4.1) and cTCD are by far more sensitive than
cTTE for detecting a right-to-left (R-L) shunt. For instance, in a recent
study, with cTCD we detected a R-L shunt in 47% of MA patients, but with
cTTE the detection rate was only 11% [6]. cTCD causes less discomfort for
the patient than cTEE, but lacks definitive proof that a shunt is due to PFO.
If necessary, the PFO can be sized via catheter angiography.

Epidemiology

PFO in the general population
A PFO can be found in about 25% of the general population (Table 4.1) [7].
The incidence and size of PFOs were studied in 965 hearts collected at
autopsy [8]. The overall prevalence was 27.3%, with equal prevalence in men
and women. Frequency decreased with age from 34.3% during the first three
decades of life, to 25.4% during the fourth through eighth decades, and to
20.2% during the ninth and tenth decades. The great majority of PFOs were
between 1 mm and 10 mm in diameter, with a mean of 4.9 mm. Diameter
increased from 3.4 mm in the first decade to 5.8 mm in the 10th decade of
life. A second autopsy study of 500 consecutive adults in which death was
due to cardiovascular disease identified a PFO in 14.6% of specimens [9,10].

PFO in migraineurs
There is an increased prevalence of PFO in migraineurs (Table 4.1).
Multiple studies using varying methods of PFO detection
(echocardiography, TCD) have supported this association. PFO is found in

Table 4.1 Prevalence of patent foramen ovale (PFO) in migraineurs compared to healthy controls.

Study	Method	Migraine with aura	Migraine without aura	Controls
Hagen et al. 1984 [8]	Autopsy	nd	nd	254/956 (27%)
Meissner et al. 1999 [10]	TEE	nd	nd	149/581 (26%)
Del Sette et al. 1998 [54]	TCD	18/44 (41%)	nd	8/50 (16%)
Anzola et al. 1999 [11]	TCD	54/113 (48%)	12/53 (23%)	5/25 (20%)
Domitzr et al. 2004 [12]	TCD	33/62 (53%)	15/60 (25%)	16/65 (25%)
Schwerzmann et al. 2005 [26]	TEE	44/93 (47%)	nd	16/93 (17%)
Total		149/312 (48%)	27/113 (24%)	448/1770 (25%)

TCD, transcranial Doppler ultrasound; TEE, transesophageal echocardiography; nd, not determined.
Reproduced from Schoenen et al. [7] with permission from Revue Médicale de Liège.

about 40–70% of people with migraine [11–16]. According to a recent systematic review, the odds ratio (OR) of a patient with migraine having a PFO is 2.5 [95% confidence interval (CI) 2.01–3.08] as compared to a patient without migraine [17].

The increased prevalence of PFO in migraine is attributable to migraineurs with aura. Although patients with migraine without aura have been studied less extensively, there does not seem to be an increased prevalence of PFO in this patient group.

The prevalence of PFO in migraineurs with aura ranges from approximately 41% to 72% [11–16]. Pooling results from several studies, the prevalence of PFO in migraineurs with aura is 54% [18]. The prevalence of PFO in migraineurs without aura ranges from approximately 16% to 34%, with a pooled prevalence of 23%, similar to the prevalence of PFO in the general non-migraine population [13,15,18].

Migraine in the general population

Migraine is a common disorder, with a lifetime prevalence of 25% in women and 8% in men, and a one-year prevalence of 18% in women and 6% in men [19,20]. Approximately one-third of people with migraine have at least an occasional aura [21]. There is a genetic propensity toward migraine, which is estimated to be superior to environmental factors in determining phenotypic expression in MA, but equal to them in migraine without aura.

Migraine in people with PFO

There is an increased prevalence of migraine in people with a PFO. The point prevalence of migraine ranges from 20% to 65% in this subject population [22–28]. The odds ratio for migraine in the presence of PFO has been estimated at 5.1 (95% CI = 4.67–5.59) [11].

The point prevalence of MA among those with PFO ranges from 13% to 50% [22–28]. The pooled prevalence from several studies is 27%, significantly higher than the expected 4% in the general population [18]. The odds ratio for MA among those with PFO is estimated at 3.2 (95% CI = 2.38–4.17) [17].

The presence of PFO does not seem to be associated with an increased prevalence of migraine without aura. The point prevalence of migraine without aura among those with PFO ranges from 3% to 25%, with a pooled prevalence of 10%, similar to that expected in the general population [22–28].

Migraine is more commonly found in the presence of a large PFO with more active right-to-left shunts [16,23,28–34].

Nature of the association between PFO and migraine

It is unclear if PFO and migraine are causally or coincidentally linked. Migraine is a complex disorder that likely has an equally complex underlying pathophysiology. It is possible that PFO could be causally related to migraine in some patients and not in others. Subgroup analyses of migraineurs with and without aura need to be completed to determine if this is true. Subgroups that may be more likely to have a causal link include: those with atypical neurologic auras, those with hypercoagulable states, those with larger PFOs, and those with more active right-to-left shunting. It is also possible that a PFO may act as a migraine trigger rather than a cause. In other words, right-to-left shunt may trigger migraine only in those people otherwise predisposed toward migraine headaches (genetic predisposition, underlying neuronal dysexcitability, propensity toward trigeminal activation, etc.). If so, this could help to explain why some patients with PFO have migraine while others do not, and why PFO closure may result in reduction in headache frequency without complete resolution.

Evidence for a causal relationship

There are several theories as to how PFO could predispose to MA episodes (Figure 4.2). Right-to-left shunting allows for paradoxical embolism of particulate material that would normally be filtered out in the lungs. These emboli may then reach the central nervous system and cause ischemia or in some other way trigger cortical spreading depression (CSD). It has been shown in animal models of CSD that depolarization of small areas of cortex can initiate the spreading wave of depolarization of neurons and glial cells characteristic of CSD [35], and that experimental microemboli may induce CSD without producing infarcts [36]. In addition, CSD has been shown to occur in the setting of acute cerebral infarct [37]. Consistent with this theory, it has been proposed that the increased prevalence of white matter (WM) hyperintensities often seen in migraineurs with aura could be secondary to small paradoxical emboli. However, there is at present no proof of a correlation between MRI WM lesions and the presence or the grade of a PFO. For instance, we found a similar 22% incidence of MRI WM lesions in MA patients whether they had or not a R-L shunt on TCD [6].

Circulatory bypass of the lungs allows for greater concentrations of serotonin to reach the central nervous system. The lungs, containing monoamine oxidase, are responsible for filtering 80–95% of venous

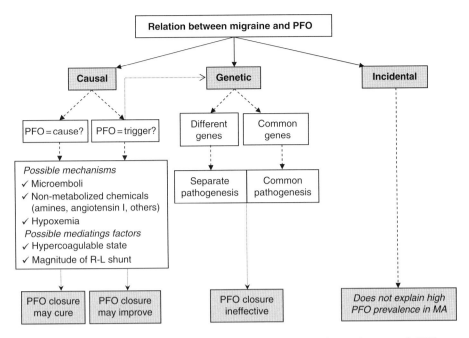

Figure 4.2 Synopsis of hypotheses on the relation between migraine and patent foramen ovale (PFO).

serotonin and other amines [3]. Serotonin has been implicated as a contributor in triggering the migraine attack [38], but its precise role is not understood. During a migraine, plasma serotonin levels increase and there is increased urinary serotonin metabolite [39,40]. In addition, brain synthesis of serotonin is increased during the attack, while it is below normal between attacks [41]. Thus, if one assumes that the ictal increase in serotonin turnover is primary and not secondary, it is feasible to theorize that elevated concentrations of arterial serotonin could trigger migraine headaches. Another circulating substance that is metabolized in the lungs is angiotensin I, which is transformed into angiotensin II by angiotensin-converting enzyme (ACE). Angiotensin I is supposed to have few biological activities, but it is not known if this also applies to subjects with genetic modifications of its metabolism or receptor. Interestingly, there is evidence, though conflicting, that the DD ACE gene polymorphism, which is associated with higher ACE levels, may increase migraine susceptibility and endothelial dysfunction [42].

The 'dose–response' relationship between PFO and migraine further supports a causal relationship. According to a recent study [43], the prevalence of PFO might be higher in patients suffering from chronic migraine than in healthy subjects and in patients suffering episodic migraine without aura, but this was not confirmed in another multicenter study [44] where prevalence of R-L shunts was in the higher range of that reported in controls. The difference could chiefly be due to the subgroup of patients who also have MA attacks and in whom R-L shunts are more prevalent. As discussed, a better established finding is that larger shunts are more commonly associated with migraine than are smaller shunts [15,23,28,30,33,34]. Larger shunts, allowing for greater volume of blood to pass directly from the venous to arterial circulation, may be associated with higher numbers of paradoxical emboli and greater concentrations of serotonin reaching the central nervous system.

Immediately following PFO closure there may be an increased incidence of MA attacks, a phenomenon supporting a causal link between PFO and migraine. It has been suggested that this increased risk in the first few weeks following PFO closure relates to formation of thrombus on the left atrial surface of the PFO occlusion device or perhaps to liberation of vasoactive substances [45]. Further supporting the theory of an embolic etiology, the frequency and severity of aura attacks following PFO closure are reduced by addition of clopidogrel therapy to daily aspirin [46]. In addition, migraine aura may rarely be precipitated during transcranial Doppler and echocardiogram bubble studies, presumably from the passage of bubbles of agitated saline to the CNS [47].

In further support of a triggering or causal relationship between PFO and migraine, extracardiac right-to-left shunts are associated with an increased prevalence of migraine. A study of 124 subjects with hereditary hemorrhagic telangiectasia (HHT), the most common cause of pulmonary arteriovenous malformations (AVMs), found 38% to have a history of migraine, 81% of whom had MA [48]. HHT subjects with pulmonary AVMs were at increased odds of having migraine, with an odds ratio of 2.4 (95% CI = 1.1–5.5, $p = 0.04$). A second study of pulmonary AVMs found 45% of such patients to have migraine, significantly higher than that expected in the general population [49]. Retrospective data collection regarding changes in migraine patterns following embolization of these pulmonary AVMs suggested significant benefit, similar to that seen in retrospective reports of PFO closure. The prevalence of migraine decreased from 45% to 34.5% after embolization ($p = 0.01$) and the prevalence of MA decreased from 33% to 19% ($p = 0.002$). In those who continued to have migraine, there was a non-significant decrease in the severity of attacks.

Given that not all people with PFO have migraine, if there is a causal or triggering relationship between the two, it can be presumed that the presence of other factors mediates this relationship. Mediating factors may include: genetic predisposition to migraine, underlying hypercoagulable states, and magnitude of right-to-left shunt.

There is some evidence to suggest that cardiac disease, even in the absence of right-to-left shunt, predisposes to migraine headache [50]. Questionnaires were employed to determine the prevalence of migraine in 395 patients with congenital heart disease and 252 sex-matched controls with acquired cardiovascular disease. The prevalence of migraine was 45% in those with congenital heart disease as compared to 11% in controls ($p < 0.001$). The prevalence of migraine was 52% among those with right-to-left shunt, 44% in those with left-to-right shunt, and 38% in those with congenital heart disease but no shunt. The high frequency of migraine in those with no shunt suggests that cardiac mechanisms other than just right-to-left shunt may contribute to the presence of migraine.

Evidence for a coincidental relationship

The association between PFO and migraine may be coincidental, without there being a causal link. The fact that no correlation was found between migraine frequency [6] and presence of PFO, or its size [51], does not support a causal relationship.

A few studies have now suggested that PFO and MA are coinherited in some families. Wilmshurst and colleagues studied 71 relatives of 20 probands with large PFOs or atrial septal defects [52]. Inheritance of atrial shunts showed an autosomal dominant pattern. When the proband had atrial shunt and MA, 71% of the first-degree relatives with a significant shunt had MA as compared to 21% of those without a significant shunt ($p < 0.02$). The investigators concluded that there is dominant inheritance of atrial shunts, which is linked to inheritance of MA in some families.

Results of the Shunt-Associated Migraine study support the assertion of a possible coinheritance of migraine and PFO. Seventy-six percent of subjects with shunt-associated migraine had a family history of migraine as compared to 66% of migraineurs without shunt ($p = 0.045$) [53].

It has been theorized that PFO and migraine could be associated yet not causally related due to common development of the endocardium, endothelium and platelets. Abnormal development of the endocardium could result in PFO, while abnormal development of endothelium and platelets could predispose to migraine [54].

Management

PFO closure and migraine: the evidence so far

Multiple retrospective studies suggest improvements in migraine patterns following closure of PFO [24–27,29,32,45,55,56]. However, these data have significant limitations and are thus not conclusive. The retrospective studies have served as an important base upon which to develop prospective, randomized, sham-controlled trials of PFO closure for migraine.

In these retrospective analyses, approximately 50% of migraineurs both with and without aura reported complete headache resolution following PFO closure. An additional 25% reported improvement in migraine patterns. Thus, three-quarters of migraineurs in these analyses benefited from PFO closure. Interestingly, benefit was equal among migraineurs with and without aura (Table 4.2) although MA patients may be 4.5 times more likely to experience post-closure relief than migraine without aura patients [57]. In the latter study it was found, moreover, that migraine relief may occur despite residual R-L shunt after the procedure. Positive results of such a magnitude have led to significant discussion and study of the PFO-migraine association. However, these results need to be interpreted in light of their limitations.

First, as mentioned, all of these studies have collected at least part of the data in a retrospective fashion. This introduces the possibility of significant recall bias. In some studies, patients were asked to recall their

Table 4.2 Outcome of patent foramen ovale (PFO) closure in retrospective studies of patients with migraine with aura (MA) and patients with migraine without aura (MO).

Study	Migraine type	Disappearence	Amelioration	Disappearance/ amelioration	No change
Wilmshurst et al. 2000 [45]	All migraines	10/21 (48%)	8/21 (38%)	18/21 (86%)	3/21 (14%)
	With aura	7/16 (44%)	8/16 (50%)	15/16 (94%)	1/16 (6%)
	Without aura	3/5 (60%)	0/5 (0%)	3/5 (60%)	2/5 (40%)
Morandi et al. 2003 [27]	Migraines	5/17 (29%)	10/17 (59%)	15/17 (88%)	2/17 (12%)
Schwerzmann et al. 2004 [26]	All migraines	NA	NA	35/43 (81%)	8/43 (19%)
	With aura	NA	NA	26/33 (79%)	7/33 (21%)
	Without aura	NA	NA	9/10 (90%)	1/10 (10%)
Azarbal et al. 2005 [55]	All migraines	19/30 (63%)	5/30 (17%)	24/30 (80%)	6/30 (20%)
	With aura	15/20 (75%)	1/20 (5%)	16/20 (80%)	4/20 (20%)
	Without aura	4/10 (40%)	4/10 (40%)	8/10 (80%)	2/10 (20%)
Post et al. 2004 [25]	All migraines	13/22 (59%)	NA	13/22 (59%)?	?
	With aura	7/10 (70%)	NA	7/10 (70%)?	?
	Without aura	6/12 (50%)	NA	6/12 (50%)?	?
Reisman et al. 2005 [24]	Migraines	28/50 (56%)	7/50 (14%)	35/50 (70%)	15/50 (30%)
Giardini et al. 2006 [56]	With aura	29/35 (83%)	3/35 (8.5%)	32/35 (91%)	3/35 (8,5%)
Kimmelstiel et al. 2007 [32]	All migraines	NA	NA	29/41 (71%)	12/41 (29%)
Total	All migraines	62/118 (53%)	30/118 (25%)	202/259 (78%)	49/237 (19%)
	With aura	22/36 (61%)	9/36 (25%)	96/114 (84%)	15/104 (14%)
	Without aura	7/15 (47%)	4/17 (24%)	26/37 (70%)	5/25 (20%)

Adapted from Schoenen et al. [7].

headache patterns for several years or more, a task that is difficult for even the most astute migraine patient. Second, it is not clear that the patients in these studies are representative of the general population of migraine patients. The majority of patients in the retrospective studies were undergoing PFO closure due to paradoxical embolism or decompression illness. This sample of patients with presumed symptomatic right-to-left shunt may be quite different from the usual migraine patient with an otherwise asymptomatic PFO. Third, there were not adequate control groups in any of these studies. Although a comparison group was used in several of the studies, a true control group was absent from all of them. The true control group, like those being used in the prospective trials, consists of subjects undergoing sham PFO closure followed by antiplatelet therapy. Although the beneficial effect of antiplatelets on migraine patterns is likely to be minimal, the placebo effect of PFO closure in the presence of any expectation of benefit is likely quite large. Fourth, headache outcomes were often measured qualitatively instead of quantitatively. For example, some studies placed patients into an 'improved' category without specific definition of improvement.

The first prospective randomized sham-controlled trial of PFO closure for the treatment of migraine is the MIST-I (Migraine in StarFlex Technology) trial [58]. Enrolled subjects had MA, at least five migraine days per month, at least seven headache-free days per month, and had failed to respond to at least two classes of standard migraine prophylactic medications. One hundred and forty-seven subjects with moderate or large PFO detected by transthoracic echocardiogram were randomized 1:1 to PFO closure or sham procedure. All subjects were treated with aspirin and clopidogrel for 3 months following the procedure. The *a priori* primary end-point was complete migraine resolution at 4–6 months post-intervention in 40% of those in the PFO closure arm. The study failed to meet this primary outcome by a large margin. Three subjects in each treatment arm had migraine resolution. Secondary end-points, such as reduction in attack frequency or in disability, were likewise not reached. Only when two patients with daily headaches, considered as outliers, were excluded, was there a significant reduction in total migraine headache days in the implant group. Device/procedure-related adverse events in the PFO closure group were as follows: cardiac tamponade ($n = 1$), pericardial effusion ($n = 1$), retroperitoneal bleed ($n = 1$), bleeding at the puncture site ($n = 1$), atrial fibrillation ($n = 2$) and atypical chest pain ($n = 2$).

Current recommendations for PFO in a patient with migraine

Based on currently available data, migraine is not an indication for PFO evaluation, except for research purposes. Furthermore, since the effects of PFO closure on migraine patterns are not defined, migraine is not an indication for PFO closure. Patients interested in PFO closure for treatment of migraine should be referred for possible inclusion in one of the prospective sham-controlled trials. Although the risks of PFO closure in an otherwise healthy patient are small, they can be significant. Currently, until more information is gathered from prospective trials, these risks outweigh any theorized benefit. Unless properly designed, sham-controlled clinical trials of PFO closure for migraine conclusively show benefit, PFO closure should not be recommended for the treatment of migraine.

Questions to be answered

Migraine characteristics predicting PFO presence

Tembl et al. hypothesized that migraine headache causally related to right-to-left shunt would be more likely triggered by maneuvers that transiently increase the magnitude of shunting (Valsalva maneuvers) [16]. Seventy-two migraineurs with aura and 31 migraineurs without aura were studied. Surveys were used to identify migraine triggers, and transcranial Doppler ultrasound with injection of agitated saline was employed for the diagnosis of shunt. Valsalva maneuvers were reported as migraine triggers in 45.8% of migraineurs with aura and in 38.7% of migraineurs without aura. Large shunts were more common in those reporting Valsalva triggers (40%)

as compared to those with absence of these triggers (12.7%), yielding an odds ratio of 2.5 (95% CI = 1.01–6.11, p = 0.032). These data suggest that Valsalva provocation of right-to-left shunt may be associated with migraine attacks in those with large shunts. Unfortunately, differences between those with and without shunt were not great enough to consider Valsalva triggering of migraine as an important predictor of right-to-left shunt presence.

The Shunt-Associated Migraine (SAM) study examined whether there were clinical features of migraine in those with right-to-left shunt that were distinct from migraine headaches in subjects without shunt [53]. Among 460 MA subjects enrolled, 42% had a right-to-left shunt and 58% had no shunt. All subjects underwent medical history, neurologic examination, brain MRI, saline contrast-enhanced transcranial Doppler ultrasound, screening for coagulation abnormalities, and transthoracic echocardiogram screening for other cardiac abnormalities. Migraine features investigated included: family history of headache, age at migraine onset, duration and characteristics of aura, migraine frequency, migraine severity, triggers, and types of abortive medications used. Unfortunately, none of the data collected adequately differentiated shunt-associated migraine from migraine not associated with shunt. However, statistical differences were found, with shunt-associated migraine subjects more frequently having a family history of migraine (76% vs 66%, p = 0.045) and more frequently having sensory symptoms during aura (51% vs 41%, p = 0.031). Based upon the parameters measured, this study suggests that shunt-associated migraine cannot be differentiated from migraine unassociated with shunt via clinical features alone.

Given that large shunts are associated with MA more often than small shunts, some investigators have queried whether large shunts are associated with more 'severe' migraine than those with smaller shunts. Gori and colleagues studied 30 MA subjects who had right-to-left shunt on transcranial Doppler ultrasound and confirmed by transesophageal echocardiogram [51]. No correlation was found between the degree of shunting and the age of onset of migraine, annual frequency of headaches, or duration of the aura phase. Although it is possible that this study was underpowered to detect a difference between groups, it serves as early evidence for a lack of an association between the degree of right-to-left shunting and several clinical measurements of migraine severity. In another study [59] looking for correlations between clinical features of MA and R-L shunts, prevalence, but not shunt degree, was greater in patients with atypical auras (19/24 patients) characterized by long duration, sudden onset or onset during headache, compared to those with typical auras (19/41). We found a comparable prevalence of large R-L whether patients had auras with strictly visual (13%) or additional neurologic symptoms (15%) [6].

Stroke, deep white matter lesions, migraine and PFO
The role of PFO in explaining the increased risk of stroke and deep WM lesions in migraine patients has been questioned. Theoretically, the increased risk of these lesions in migraineurs could be attributable to paradoxical emboli conveyed via right-to-left shunts. Cerebellar vascular

border-zone infarcts are more common in migraine patients than controls, with an odds ratio for these lesions of 7.1 (95% CI = 0.9–55) [60]. The highest risk is found among migraineurs with aura who have more frequent attacks (OR 15.8; 95% CI = 1.8–140) [60]. Deep WM lesions are more common in women migraineurs than controls (OR 2.1; 95% CI = 1.0–4.1) [50]. Similar to the relationship between cerebellar strokes and migraine, migraineurs with more frequent attacks are even more likely to have deep WM hyperintensities as compared to controls (OR 2.6; 95% CI = 1.2–5.7). It has been theorized that these infarcts and possibly these deep WM lesions are secondary to migraine attack-related hypoperfusion and/or embolism [61].

A few studies have indirectly supported a relationship between PFO, migraine and stroke. Although not typical of the lesions commonly found in migraineurs, there have been case reports of 'migrainous infarction' from paradoxical embolism via PFO [62]. Further studies are required to explore this possible relationship.

The association between right-to-left shunt and WM lesions in migraineurs with aura has been investigated by studying 87 MA subjects via transcranial Doppler ultrasound and brain MRI [63]. Right-to-left shunts were detected in 45% of the subjects; WM lesions were seen in 61%. None of the subjects had diffusion-weighted hyperintense lesions suggestive of acute stroke. There was no significant difference in the presence, number or volume of WM lesions in the subjects with right-to-left shunt as compared to those without. These data held even when considering only large shunts. This finding was replicated in two larger studies of 185 [64] and 114 [6] MA patients. In the former, which is part of the SAM study, MRI WM lesion load was similar in patients with or without a R-L shunt, lesions in deep WM being even less pronounced in patients with a R-L shunt ($p < 0.045$). We have found the same 22% incidence of MRI WM lesions whether a R-L shunt was detected or not; there was, however, a trend for a greater number of lesions in subjects with large shunts, but this was attributed to two patients with ≥20 lesions [6]. Finally, in one study the risk of cerebral lesions being detected on MRI was even smaller in patients with a R-L shunt compared to those who had none (OR 0.589; 95% CI = 0.193–1.799) [65]. All these studies certainly argue against the notion that shunting of emboli via PFO may explain the increased prevalence of WM lesions in patients with migraine.

Hypercoagulable state, PFO and migraine

It is theorized that patients with PFO that results in migraine may have an increased frequency of underlying hypercoagulable disorders. For instance, in a retrospective study of 131 patients who underwent transcatheter PFO closure, those who suffered from MA ($n = 35$) had a higher prevalence of thrombophilia [56]. In the presence of hypercoagulability, it may be more likely that small thrombi would form, perhaps in the PFO tunnel, and thus embolize to the central nervous system triggering migraine. This possibility was investigated in 460 subjects, 42% of whom had right-to-left shunt [53]. Screening for coagulation abnormalities included tests for plasma levels of protein C, protein S and homocysteine, activated protein

C resistance, factor II and V Leiden, presence of antiphospholipid antibodies, and methylenetetrahydrofolate reductase gene polymorphisms. Contrary to the hypothesis, migraineurs with shunts were less likely to have a coagulation abnormality (23% vs 37%, $p = 0.011$). The investigators suggest that this finding might be genetically determined in association with the persistence of the foramen ovale or might reflect an increased susceptibility of people with PFO to develop headache even with minor or absent hypercoagulable states. Similarly, Marchione et al. [59] found no difference in thrombophilic factors between subjects with typical or atypical aura whether a R-L shunt was present or not.

PFO closure for migraine treatment

Completion and results from additional prospective sham-controlled trials of PFO closure for migraine are needed to understand a potential role of closure for migraine. Several such studies are currently enrolling. However, enrollment has proved challenging in North America. The MIST-II trial as well as other planned trials were prematurely closed for enrollment, reportedly due to high study costs related to slow enrollment.

Clinical summary points

- Patent foramen ovale is more common in people who have migraine with aura.
- Migraine with aura is more frequent in people who have a patent foramen ovale.
- It is unclear if there is a causal or coincidental relationship between migraine with aura and patent foramen ovale.
- There seems to be no correlation between PFO and severity of migraine or MRI white matter lesion load.
- The role of patent foramen ovale closure for the treatment of migraine is not yet defined.
- At this time, given the strength and quality of existing data, the usual evaluation of a patient with migraine does not include evaluation for presence of a patent foramen ovale.
- At this time, treatment of migraine aura and/or headache is not an indication for patent foramen ovale closure.
- Ongoing randomised controlled trials may determine which subgroups of migraine with aura patients benefit from PFO closure.

Case report (continued)

The 34-year-old migraine patient described previously was finally treated with lamotrigine at slowly increasing doses up to 150 mg/day in addition to amitriptyline. After 2 months her migraine with aura attacks had resolved completely, but she still had one attack without aura per week, which she treats with a triptan-non-steroidal anti-inflammatory drug (NSAID) combination. She considered that this was an acceptable situation.

References

1 Langholz D, Louie EK, Konstadt SN, Rao TL, Scanlon PJ. Transesophageal echocardiographic demonstration of distinct mechanisms for right to left shunting across a patent foramen ovale in the absence of pulmonary hypertension. J Am Coll Cardiol 1991;18:1112–17.

2 Sukernik MR, Bennett-Guerrero E. The incidental finding of a patent foramen ovale during cardiac surgery: should it always be repaired? A core review. Anesth Analg 2007;105:602–10.

3 Gillis CN, Pitt BR. The fate of circulating amines within the pulmonary circulation. Ann Rev Physiol 1982;44:269–81.

4 Jauss M, Zanette E. Detection of right-to-left shunt with ultrasound contrast agent and transcranial Doppler sonography. Cerebrovasc Dis 2000;10: 490–6.

5 Spencer MP, Moehring MA, Jesurum J, Gray WA, Olsen JV, Reisman M. Power m-mode transcranial Doppler for diagnosis of patent foramen ovale and assessing transcatheter closure. J Neuroimaging 2004;14:342–9.

6 Shalchian S, Gérardy PY, Damas F, Schoenen J. Prevalence of patent foramen ovale and MRI white matter lesions in migraine with aura: a cross-sectional study. Cephalalgia 2009;29:120.

7 Schoenen J, Burette P, Materne P. Patent foramen ovale and migraine: incidental or causal association? Rev Med Liège 2006; 61:9–15.

8 Hagen PT, Scholz DG, Edwards WD. Incidence and size of patent foramen ovale during the first 10 decades of life: an autopsy study of 965 normal hearts. Mayo Clin Proc 1984;59:17–20.

9 Penther P. Patent foramen ovale: an anatomical study. A propos of 500 consecutive autopsies. Arch Mal Coeur Vaiss 1994;87:15–21.

10 Meissner I, Whisnant JP, Khandheria BK, et al. Prevalence of potential risk factors for stroke assessed by transesophageal echocardiography and carotid ultrasonography: the SPARC study. Stroke Prevention: Assessment of Risk in a Community. Mayo Clin Proc 1999;74:862–9.

11 Anzola GP, Magoni MD, Guindani M, Rozzini L, Dalla Volta GD. Potential source of cerebral embolism in migraine with aura. A transcranial Doppler study. Neurology 1999;52:1622–5.

12 Domitrz I, Mieszkowski J, Kwiecinski H. The prevalence of patent foramen ovale in patients with migraine. Neurol Neurochir Pol 2004;38: 89–92.

13 Dalla Volta G, Guindani M, Zavarise P, Griffini S, Pezzini A, Padovani A. Prevalence of patent foramen ovale in a large series of patients with migraine with aura, migraine without aura and cluster headache, and relationship with clinical phenotype. J Headache Pain 2005;6:328–30.

14 Ferrarini G, Malferrari G, Zucco R, Gaddi O, Norina M, Pini LA. High prevalence of patent foramen ovale in migraine with aura. J Headache Pain 2005;6:71–6.

15 Carod-Artal FJ, da Silveira Ribeiro L, Braga H, Kummer W, Mesquita HM, Vargas AP. Prevalence of patent foramen ovale in migraine patients with and without aura compared with stroke patients. A transcranial Doppler study. Cephalalgia 2006;26:934–9.

16 Tembl J, Lago A, Sevilla T, Solis P, Vilchez J. Migraine, patent foramen ovale and migraine triggers. J Headache Pain 2007;8:7–12.

17 Schwedt TJ, Demaerschalk BM, Dodick DW. Patent foramen ovale and migraine: a quantitative systematic review. Cephalalgia 2008;28:531–40.

18 Schwedt TJ, Dodick DW. Patent foramen ovale and migraine – bringing closure to the subject. Headache 2006;46:663–71.

19 Stewart WF, Lipton RB, Celentano DO et. al. Prevalence of migraine headache in the United States: relation to age, income, race, and other socioeconomic factors. JAMA 1992;267:64–9.

20 Lipton RB, Stewart WF, Diamond S, Diamond ML, Reed M. Prevalence and burden of migraine in the United States: data from the American Migraine Study II. Headache 2001;41:646–57.

21 Rasmussen BK. Epidemiology of headache. Cephalalgia 2001;21:774–7.

22 Sztajzel R, Genoud D, Roth S, Mermillod B, Le Floch-Rohr J. Patent foramen ovale, a possible cause of symptomatic migraine: a study of 74 patients with acute ischemic stroke. Cerebrovasc Dis 2002;13:102–6.

23 Wilmshurst P, Pearson M, Nightingale S. Re-evaluation of the relationship between migraine and persistent foramen ovale and other right-to-left shunts. Clin Sci (Lond) 2005;108:365–7.

24 Reisman M, Christofferson RD, Jesurum J, et al. Migraine headache relief after transcatheter closure of patent foramen ovale. J Am Coll Cardiol 2005;45:493–5.

25 Post MC, Thijs V, Herroelen L, Budts WI. Closure of a patent foramen ovale is associated with a decrease in prevalence of migraine. Neurology 2004;62:1439–40.

26 Schwerzmann M, Wiher S, Nedeltchev K, et al. Percutaneous closure of patent foramen ovale reduces the frequency of migraine attacks. Neurology 2004;62:1399–401.

27 Morandi E, Anzola GP, Angeli S, Melzi G, Onorato E. Transcatheter closure of patent foramen ovale: a new migraine treatment? J Interv Cardiol 2003;16:39–42.

28 Wilmshurst P, Nightingale S. Relationship between migraine and cardiac and pulmonary right-to-left shunts. Clin Sci (Lond) 2001;100:215–20.

29 Anzola GP, Frisoni GB, Morandi E, Casilli F, Onorato E. Shunt-associated migraine responds favorably to atrial septal repair: a case-control study. Stroke 2006;37:430–4.

30 Anzola GP, Morandi E, Casilli F, Onorato E. Different degrees of right-to-left shunting predict migraine and stroke: data from 420 patients. Neurology 2006;66:765–7.

31 Wilmshurst P, Nightingale S, Pearson M, Morrison L, Walsh K. Relation of atrial shunts to migraine in patients with ischemic stroke and peripheral emboli. Am J Cardiol 2006;98:831–3.

32 Kimmelstiel C, Gange C, Thaler D. Is patent foramen ovale closure effective in reducing migraine symptoms? A controlled study. Catheter Cardiovasc Interv 2007;69:740–6.

33 Schwerzmann M, Nedeltchev K, Lagger F, et al. Prevalence and size of directly detected patent foramen ovale in migraine with aura. Neurology 2005;65:1415–18.

34 Jesurum JT, Fuller CJ, Velez CA, et al. Migraineurs with patent foramen ovale have larger right-to-left shunt despite similar atrial septal characteristics. J Headache Pain 2007;8:209–16.

35 James MF, Smith MI, Bockhorst KH et al. Cortical spreading depression in the gyrencephalic feline brain studied by magnetic resonance imaging. J Physiol 1999;519;415–25.

36 Nozari A, Dilekoz E, Sukhotinsky I et al. Microemboli may link spreading depression, migraine aura, and patent foramen ovale. Ann Neurol 2010;67:221–9.

37 Wang Z, Li P, Luo W, Chen S, Luo Q. Peri-infarct temporal changes in intrinsic optical signal during spreading depression in focal ischemic rat cortex. Neurosci Lett 2007;424:133–8.

38 Schwedt TJ. Serotonin and migraine: the latest developments. Cephalalgia 2007;27:1301–7.

39 Ferrari MD, Odink J, Tapparelli C, Van Kempen GMJ, Pennings EJM, Bruyn GW. Serotonin metabolism in migraine. Neurology 1989;39:1239–42.

40 Sicuteri F, Testi A, Anselmi B. Biochemical investigations in headache: increase in the hydroxyindoleacetic acid excretion during migraine attacks. Int Arch Allergy 1961;19:55–8.

41 Sakai Y, Dobson C, Diksic M, Aubé M, Hamel E. Sumatriptan normalizes the migraine attack-related increase in brain serotonin synthesis. Neurology 2008;70;431–9.

42 Tietjen GE, Herial NA, Utley C, White L, Yerga-Woolwine S, Joe B. Association of von Willebrand factor activity with ACE I/D and MTHFR C677T polymorphisms in migraine. Cephalalgia 2009;29:960–8.

43 Nahas SJ, Young WB, Terry R et al. Right-to-left shunt is common in chronic migraine. Cephalalgia 2010;30:535–42.

44 Shalchian S, Ashina M, Guo S, Küper M, Katsarava Z, Schoenen J. Left shunt prevalence on ctcd in chronic migraine with or without medication overuse headache: a cross-sectional study. Acta Neurol Belg 2010;110(Suppl. 1):46.

45 Wilmshurst PT, Nightingale S, Walsh KP et. al. Effect on migraine of closure of cardiac right-to-left shunts to prevent recurrence of decompression illness or stroke for haemodynamic reasons. Lancet 2000;356:1648–51.

46 Wilmshurst PT, Nightingale S, Walsh KP, Morrison WL. Clopidogrel reduces migraine with aura after transcatheter closure of persistent foramen ovale and atrial septal defects. Heart 2005;91:1173–5.

47 Dinia L, Roccatagliata L, Bonzano L, Finocchi C, Del Sette M. Diffusion MRI during migraine with aura attack associated with diagnostic microbubbles injection in subjects with large PFO. Headache 2007;47:1455–6.

48 Thenganatt J, Schneiderman J, Hyland RH, Edmeads J, Mandzia JL, Faughnan ME. Migraines linked to intrapulmonary right-to-left shunt. Headache 2006;46:439–43.

49 Post MC, Thijs V, Schonewille WJ, et al. Embolization of pulmonary arteriovenous malformations and decrease in prevalence of migraine. Neurology 2006;66:202–5.

50 Truong T, Slavin L, Kashani R et. al. Prevalence of migraine headaches in patients with congenital heart disease. Am J Cardiol 2008;101:396–400.

51 Gori S, Morelli N, Fannucchi S, et al. The extent of right-to-left shunt fails to correlate with severity of clinical picture in migraine with aura. Neurol Sci 2006;27:14–17.

52 Wilmshurst PT, Pearson MJ, Nightingale S, Walsh KP, Morrison WL. Inheritance of persistent foramen ovale and atrial septal defects and the relation to familial migraine with aura. Heart 2004;90:1315–20.

53 Anzola GP, Meneghetti G, Zanferrari C, Adami A, Dinia L, Del Sette M, for the SAM Study Group. Is migraine associated with right-to-left shunt a separate disease? Results of the SAM study. Cephalalgia 2008;28:360–6.

54 Del Sette M, Angeli S, Leandri M et. al. Migraine with aura and right-to-left shunt on transcranial Doppler: a case-control study. Cerebrovasc Dis 1998;8:327–30.

55 Azarbal B, Tobis J, Suh W et. al. Association of interatrial shunts and migraine headaches. J Am Coll Cardiol 2005;45:489–92.

56 Giardini A, Donti A, Formigari R, et al. Transcatheter patent foramen ovale closure mitigates aura migraine headaches abolishing spontaneous right-to-left shunting. Am Heart J 2006;151:922.e1–5.

57 Jesurum JT, Fuller CJ, Kim CJ, et al. Frequency of migraine headache relief following patent foramen ovale 'closure' despite residual right-to-left shunt. Am J Cardiol 2008;102:916–20.

58 Dowson A, Mullen MJ, Peatfield R, et al. Migraine Intervention With STARFlex Technology (MIST) Trial: A prospective, multicenter, double-blind, sham-controlled trial to evaluate the effectiveness of patent foramen ovale closure with STARFlex septal repair implant to resolve refractory migraine headache. Circulation 2008;117:1397–404.

59 Marchione P, Ghiotto N, Sances G, et al. Clinical implications of patent foramen ovale in migraine with aura. Funct Neurol 2008;23:201–5.

60 Kruit MC, van Buchem MA, Hofman PAM, et al. Migraine as a risk factor for subclinical brain lesions. JAMA 2004;291:427–34.

61 Kruit MC, Launer LJ, Ferrari M, van Buchem MA. Infarcts in the posterior circulation territory in migraine. The population-based MRI CAMERA study. Brain 2005;128:2068–77.

62 Ries S, Steinke W, Neff W, Schindlmayr C, Meairs S, Hennerici M. Ischemia-induced migraine from paradoxical cardioembolic stroke. Eur Neurol 1996;36:76–8.

63 Del Sette M, Dinia L, Bonzano L, et al. White matter lesions in migraine and right-to-left shunt: a conventional and diffusion MRI study. Cephalalgia 2008;28:376–82.

64 Adami A, Rossato G, Cerini R, et al. on behalf of the SAM Study Group. Right-to-left shunt does not increase white matter lesion load in migraine with aura patients. Neurology 2008;71:101–7.

65 Ramírez-Moreno JM, Casado-Naranjo I, Gómez M, et al. Migraine with aura and patent foramen ovale. A different clinical entity? Neurologia 2008;23:503–10.

5 Comorbidity of Migraine and Epilepsy

Sheryl Haut[1,2], Shira Markowitz[2] and Richard B. Lipton[2,3]

[1] Comprehensive Epilepsy Management Center, Montefiore Medical Center, Albert Einstein College of Medicine, NY, USA

[2] Department of Neurology, Albert Einstein College of Medicine, NY, USA

[3] Department of Epidemiology and Population Health, Albert Einstein College of Medicine and Montefiore Headache Unit, NY, USA

Case presentation

Marlie, a 27-year-old woman with a history since adolescence of intractable migraine with aura, presented with the recent onset of a new type of attack. Previously her migraine attacks occurred five to eight times per week and often began with typical visual aura followed by unilateral, pulsatile headache with nausea, photophobia and phonophobia. Treatment with maximally tolerated doses of verapamil and nortriptyline reduced attack frequency, and treatment with a triptan usually relieved the acute attacks in a couple of hours.

The new-onset attacks are characterized by confusion followed by generalized stiffness and shaking. They last up to 5 minutes each, without incontinence or tongue biting. The new events are not clearly associated with headache. An electroencephalogram (EEG) did not reveal potentially epileptogenic abnormalities. Nonetheless, the clinical service thought these events might represent the new onset of a localization-related epilepsy in a patient with migraine, a new form of atypical aura without headache or non-epileptic events.

To distinguish these possibilities she was admitted for continuous video/EEG monitoring. During monitoring, while talking to a family member on the phone she reported her 'worst migraine aura in years'. The EEG revealed a rhythmic seizure discharge in the right temporo-occipital region (Figure 5.1). As the discharge evolved and spread (Figure 5.2), the patient developed a brief period of confusion during which she was unable to answer questions, followed by a generalized tonic clonic seizure. She was discharged with a diagnosis of migraine with aura and partial complex seizures with secondary generalization.

Comorbidity in Migraine, First Edition. Edited by J. Schoenen, D. W. Dodick and P. S. Sándor.
© 2011 Blackwell Publishing Ltd. Published 2011 by Blackwell Publishing Ltd.

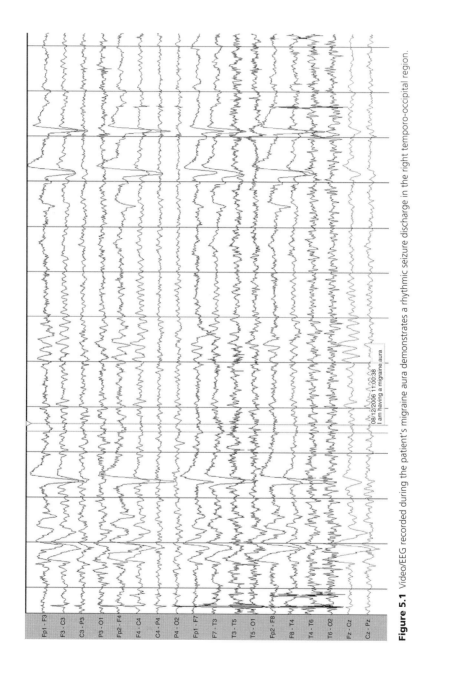

Figure 5.1 Video/EEG recorded during the patient's migraine aura demonstrates a rhythmic seizure discharge in the right temporo-occipital region.

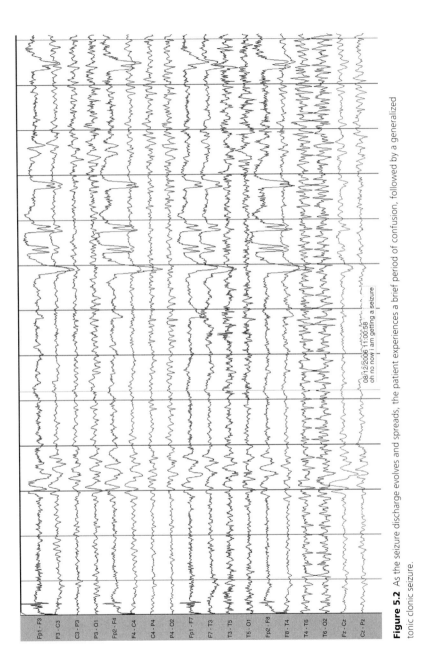

Figure 5.2 As the seizure discharge evolves and spreads, the patient experiences a brief period of confusion, followed by a generalized tonic clonic seizure.

Introduction

Migraine and epilepsy may occur in the same individuals [1] and have much in common as chronic neurologic disorders with episodic attacks (CDEA) [2]. Both migraine and epilepsy represent families of disorders, which differ in their clinical presentation, natural history and response to treatment [3–5]. These families of disorders are sometimes referred to as 'the migraines' and 'the epilepsies' to reflect the heterogeneity encompassed within each broad category. Both families of disorders have international classifications – the International Classification of Headache Disorders, 2nd edition (ICHD-2) for migraine, and the International League Against Epilepsy Classification, for epilepsy [6,7]. Both the migraines and the epilepsies are characterized by attacks of neurologic dysfunction that may include alteration of consciousness, sensory or motor manifestations, and pain as well as autonomic, gastrointestinal and psychological features. Between attacks persons with each disorder have an enduring predisposition to attacks, possibly taking the form of brain hyperexcitability.

Understanding the relationships among migraine and epilepsy is important for several reasons. As our patient history illustrates, these disorders may occur together in the same individual [8]. This occurs with a frequency much greater than by chance [9–11]. Because migraine and epilepsy travel together, diagnosis of either of these disorders should heighten the index of diagnostic suspicion for the other. Marlie's migraines make it more likely that she will also have epilepsy. However, the overlap of clinical features creates a challenge in differential diagnosis. Prior to EEG monitoring, it was possible that Marlie's new attacks might have represented a new form of aura. Migraine and epilepsy may be linked at the level of mechanism and neurobiology as both are conceptualized as disorders of brain hyperexcitability. The genetic and environmental risk factors for migraine and epilepsy overlap [9,10], while the treatments used substantially overlap but are also substantially distinct.

In this chapter, we describe the epidemiology of migraine and epilepsy and the evidence that the conditions are comorbid. We consider the pathophysiologic mechanisms that may link migraine and epilepsy as well as the genetic and environmental factors common to these disorders. Following an overview of diagnosis, we contrast the phases of attacks of migraine and epilepsy, and review the diagnosis of migraine variants most often mistaken for epilepsy. Finally, we will briefly discuss treatment considerations.

Epidemiologic connections between migraine and epilepsy

In their now classic review, Andermann and Andermann summarized studies showing that the 1-year period prevalence of epilepsy is about 0.5% in the general population; in persons with migraine, epilepsy prevalence ranged from 1% to 17%, with a median of 5.9% [1,9]. Other studies have examined this comorbidity; Marks and Ehrenberg found that of 79 of 395 patients with epilepsy, i.e. 20%, also had IHS migraine [8]. Velioglu and Özmenoglu found that among 412 adults with epilepsy, 14% had IHS migraine [12].

Ottman and Lipton examined the association between migraine and epilepsy using data from the Epilepsy Family Study of Columbia University [10,13]. Among probands with epilepsy the prevalence of migraine was 24%. In their relatives with epilepsy migraine prevalence was 26%. In relatives without epilepsy, only 15% had migraine. The incidence of migraine in persons with epilepsy was 2.4 times higher than in persons without epilepsy. Migraine risk was elevated in every subgroup of epilepsy defined by seizure type, age of onset, and etiology of epilepsy. The age of onset of epilepsy did not influence the risk of migraine.

Migraine with aura may have an even greater comorbidity with epilepsy than migraine without aura; in two recent studies, the prevalence of epilepsy in children with migraine with aura was 30%, and the incidence of new-onset seizures was recently reported to be increased in pediatric patients with migraine with aura as compared to migraine without aura [14,15]. In at least one population study, a relationship between migraine and epilepsy was not demonstrated, though the power was limited and migraine was present in 5 of 11 subjects with epilepsy [16].

Pathophysiology: mechanisms that link migraine and epilepsy

Unidirectional causal models

The mechanisms of the association between migraine and epilepsy are complex and may be multifactorial. One possibility is a simple unidirectional causal explanation. For example, migraine may increase the risk of epilepsy by inducing brain ischemia and injury. On the other hand, epilepsy may cause migraine-like headaches if the electrical activity of a seizure activates meningeal nociceptors, potentially producing ictal headaches and predisposing to interictal headaches. Ictal and post-ictal headaches with migraine-like features have been well demonstrated in up to half of patients with epilepsy [17]. If the headache is attributable to the seizure these headaches would be considered secondary headache and not migraine according to the ICHD-2, even if they have migrainous features [6,17]. If epilepsy predisposes to interictal headaches with migraine-like features, then we would consider it a risk factor for migraine.

If epilepsy predisposes to migraine and not vice versa, we would expect the incidence of migraine to increase after the onset of epilepsy, but not before it. Data from the Epilepsy Family Study and elsewhere show that there is an excess risk of migraine both before and after seizure onset, leading to the rejection of both unidirectional causal models.

Shared environmental risk factors

While it is possible that shared environmental risk factors link headache and epilepsy, this is more problematic for migraines. Migraine is defined as a primary headache disorder without a known underlying cause. Thus headaches secondary to symptomatic causes such as head injury or stroke are not classified as migraine [18], even if the headache syndrome is identical to migraine. In the Epilepsy Family Study [10], we examined the known environmental risk factors of epilepsy, including head injury, meningitis, stroke and structural brain disease [19,20]. Of these environmental risk factors for epilepsy, only head injury was associated with an increase in migraine, and it accounted for only a small proportion of the observed comorbidity.

Genetic risk factors

If shared genetic risk factors account for comorbidity, the risk of migraine should be higher in families with genetic versus non-genetic forms of epilepsy. This was not demonstrated in the family study described above [21]. Though genetic risk factors do not appear to account for the overall relationship between migraine and epilepsy, specific genetic polymorphisms, discussed below, contribute to this association.

Do migraine and epilepsy have a common brain substrate?

The pathophysiologic models of both migraine and epilepsy appear to involve an overall imbalance between neuronal excitation and inhibition [22–24]. Seizures are the manifestation of abnormal hypersynchronous discharges of cortical neurons. The neurophysiologic excitability of neurons and the communication between them rely on axonal conduction mediated by action potentials, and on signal transduction mediated by synaptic transmission [23]. Essential to these processes are ionic conductances of sodium, potassium (generation of the action potential) and calcium (synaptic release of neurotransmitter). Although the demonstration of genetic alterations in epilepsy have thus far been limited to a number of idiopathic generalized epilepsies and certain symptomatic syndromes [25], it is clear from the evidence available that alterations in ionic transmission figure prominently. Similarly, the genetics of migraine thus far have been largely described in familial hemiplegic migraine (FHM) [26], and contain very similar alterations in ion conductance. As data regarding ion channel dysfunction in epilepsy and migraine accumulate, both families of disorders are increasingly thought of as 'channelopathies' [27].

As discussed in the classification section below, both migraine and epilepsy encompass events with varying classifications and manifestations. The descriptions thus far of shared genetics between migraine and migraine refer to specific syndromes within each disorder. However, elements of the overall pathophysiologies of epilepsy and migraine show striking similarities. The development of hyperexcitable neuronal circuits in epilepsy, a process known as epileptogenesis, is complex and related to the interplay between glutamatergic (excitatory) and GABAergic (inhibitory) neurotransmitter activity [24,28]. In hyperexcitable, epileptic neuronal circuits, the characteristic end result is an imbalance between excitatory and inhibitory activity. This imbalance may be molecular and/or functional, related to changes in components that are directly involved in glutamatergic transmission, the GABAergic system, or both. Examining the pathophysiology of migraine, particularly in relation to migraine with aura, reveals a similarity in enhanced neuronal hyperexcitability and a reduced threshold to attacks [29]. It has been established that cortical spreading depression (CSD), consisting of a wave of excitation followed by a wave of inhibition that moves across the cortical mantle, is the mechanism behind migraine aura [30–32]. Studies have shown that altered concentrations of GABA (γ-aminobutyric acid), magnesium and glutamate are key factors in creating a hyperexcitable state, which sustains the propagation of CSD [33,34].

FHM genes and epilepsy

The three major loci involved in familial hemiplegic migraine (FHM; ICHD-II 1.2.4) have also been associated with epilepsy [35]. FHM is a rare autosomal dominant form of migraine characterized by hemiparesis as part of the migraine aura [6]. The three genes implicated in FHM code for a neuronal P/Q type calcium channel (*CACN1A*), for a Na+/K+ ATPase (ATP1A2) and for a sodium channel (SCN1A). Mutations in each of these genes have also been identified in various forms of epilepsy [35].

- *CACNA1A:* The FHM1 gene *CACNA1A* is located on chromosome 19 and codes for the main subunit of the CaV2.1 P/Q neuronal calcium channel [36–38]. Numerous mutations of this gene have been associated with FHM1, at least seven of which are also associated with epilepsy [35]. Epilepsy phenotypes are variable; most patients have localization-related seizures, though generalized seizures and seizures with fatal coma have been reported. Phenotypes are variable even among carriers with the same mutation and within the same family [39,40]. The mutant *CACNA1A* gene causes increased calcium influx through the CaV2.1 channel. It is thought that this alteration in the channel leads to activation of the channel in response to smaller depolarizations, which would be insufficient to open wild-type channels. The increased calcium influx may lead to enhanced glutamate release, creating a hyperexcitable state that makes the cortex more susceptible to seizures and to the spreading depression implicated in migraine aura [23,41].

- *ATP1A2:* The FHM2 gene, found on the long arm of chromosome 1 in the 1q23 region, codes for the alpha1 subunit of a Na+/K+ ATPase [42–45]. At least 10 distinct mutations in this gene have been associated with a range of seizure disorders including partial seizures, benign familial infantile convulsions andgeneralized seizures [35]. Genetic analysis of two Dutch families, one with pure FHM and one with both FHM and benign familial infantile convulsions (BFIC), identified two different mutations of *ATP1A2*. One was associated with pure FHM, the other was found in family members with FHM, BFIC or both [46]. In a recent analysis of a French family with FHM, the proband had childhood absence epilepsy as well as generalized tonic clonic seizures. Many of the migraine attacks were triggered by the generalized seizures. Interestingly, sodium valproate treated both the seizures and the FHM attacks [47]. There are examples of many other mutations in *ATP1A2* that have been found in families with FHM and epilepsy [35]. The loss of function of the Na$^+$/K$^+$ pump caused by mutations in the *ATP1A2* gene has been proposed to cause cortical depolarization by two mechanisms: (i) impaired clearance of potassium leading to elevated extracellular levels, and (ii) elevated intracellular sodium, causing increased intracellular calcium via the Na$^+$/Ca^{2+} exchanger, resembling the effect of the *CACNA1A* mutation in FHM1 [45]. In addition, the altered sodium gradient causes impaired synaptic glutamate clearance. The resulting elevated glutamate level is involved in the initiation of cortical spreading depression as well as epileptic events [22].

- *SCN1A:* A third locus for FHM was identified on chromosome 2q24 encoding the neuronal sodium channel gene *SCN1A* [48]. Mutations in the *SCN1A* gene have been identified as an important cause of a number of epilepsy syndromes for some time, and *SCN1A* mutation testing is performed in clinical pediatric epilepsy practice. Interestingly, this gene is associated with a spectrum of epilepsy severity, ranging from generalized epilepsy with febrile seizures plus type 2 (GEFS+2), typically a mild form of epilepsy, to severe myoclonic epilepsy of infancy (SMEI) [49–51]. Studies of the electrophysiology of *SCN1A* genetic mutations found in GEFS+ demonstrated impaired sodium channel inactivation and consequently a reduced threshold for action potential firing. This is believed to cause neuronal hyperexcitability creating a brain substrate that is more susceptible to seizures [52]. Similarly, the functional consequences of the sodium channel mutation in FHM were studied by introducing the FHM3 mutation into myocardial sodium channel *SCN5* (this gene is homologous to *SCN1*).This mutation was also shown to impair inactivation of sodium channels and is thought to play a role in the enhanced neuronal excitability leading to CSD [48].

It has become clear that genetic mutations in these three genes shared by migraine and epilepsy cause changes in ion concentrations and membrane potential within the neuronal network that are believed to be responsible for its hyperexcitable state. The shared pathophysiologic mechanism underlying the genetic/channelopathy aspect of migraine and epilepsy is intriguing. Although in theory genetic or environmental factors could produce these alterations, the commonality in the electrophysiologic changes in FHM and epilepsy subtype sheds light on the relationship between the two disorders as a whole.

Diagnosis and classification

For both migraine and epilepsy, each family of disorders has an internationally recognized classification system [6,7,53]. The ICHD-2 defines four primary types and 10 secondary forms [6]. Primary headaches include migraine, tension-type headache, trigeminal autonomic cephalalgias (including cluster headache) as well as a group of 'other primary headaches'. Migraine is further divided into five major categories, the two most important of which are migraine without aura (formerly common migraine) and migraine with aura (formerly classic migraine). Headache diagnosis is usually based on the retrospective reporting of attack characteristics. The results of general medical and neurologic examinations, as well as laboratory studies, are usually normal and serve to exclude other, more ominous, causes of headache.

Seizures and epileptic syndromes are classified in a somewhat similar manner, utilizing a classification system developed by the International League Against Epilepsy (ILAE) [53]. The ILAE classifies seizure types as partial (or focal with or without secondary generalization) or generalized. Epilepsy is diagnosed after the occurrence of two unprovoked seizures [54]. The etiology of epilepsy may be idiopathic, symptomatic or cryptogenic. The idiopathic epilepsies are similar to the primary headache disorders in that recurrent attacks occur without an apparent underlying cause. In these, the predominant type of seizure begins simultaneously in both cerebral hemispheres. Many forms of idiopathic generalized epilepsy have a strong genetic component; in most, neurologic function is normal. The symptomatic and cryptogenic epilepsies, like secondary headaches, are attributed to an identified or presumed underlying disorder. In these, seizures originate in one or more focal regions, although they can spread to involve the entire brain.

In addition to being comorbid, migraines and seizures have significant overlap, including similarities in ictal progression, and associated symptoms [55]. Although the shared characteristics can lead to confusion and misdiagnosis, the differentiation is typically not difficult. The most important tool in differentiating between migraine without aura and epilepsy is the history. Tables 5.1 and 5.2 present the features most useful in distinguishing them. In general, in comparison with epilepsy, attacks of migraine are more gradual in onset and of longer duration. Nausea and vomiting are more commonly associated with migraine, while prolonged confusion or lethargy after the attack favors epilepsy.

At times, differentiating migraine with aura from epilepsy can be difficult, particularly when motor manifestations are absent. The characteristics of the aura may help: the migraine aura is longer (>5 min) and the aura of epilepsy is brief (usually <1 min) [5,56,57]. In addition, the aura symptom profiles differ, and are discussed in detail below.

Correctly diagnosing and separating epilepsy and migraine can be more difficult in children since children may give incomplete descriptions of their symptoms. In addition, features useful in diagnosing epilepsy or migraine in adults may be absent or difficult to elicit in children. Hemicranial pain and visual auras occur less often in children with migraine, and the first symptoms of migraine may not even be associated with headaches [58]. Children are also less likely to experience feelings of déjà vu or to have olfactory hallucinations as part of a simple partial seizure or temporal lobe epilepsy. Furthermore, the epilepsies most commonly mistaken for migraine are childhood syndromes, as discussed below.

Table 5.1 Comparison of prodromal symptoms, ictal events and postdromes in migraine versus epilepsy.

	Migraine	Epilepsy
Prodromal symptoms	Common (60%) • Irritability, joy or sadness • Talkativeness or social withdrawal • Appetite change or anorexia • Water retention • Sleep disturbances	Less common • Heaviness, depression, irritability • GI upset • Headache in 3–11% of all patients
Ictus	Prolonged (4–72 hours) unilateral throbbing headache with associated features	Brief, self-limited (1–2 min) seizure *Exception:* status epilepticus: 30+ min
Postdrome	Impaired concentration, malaise or euphoria	• Confusion, lethargy, depressed consciousness, marked after generalized tonic clonic seizure • Up to 40% of all patients report post-ictal headache, and many are migrainous in quality

Table 5.2 Comparison of symptoms in migraine with aura versus epilepsy.

	Migraine	Epilepsy
Premonitory	Common	Often
Duration of aura	15–60 min	Brief, often <1 min
Automatisms (repetitive purposeless movements)	Unusual	Absent in aura, often present in complex partial seizures; i.e. blinking or chewing
Gastrointestinal aura	Abdominal pain (rare) Nausea (common)	'Butterflies' – rising epigastric sensation
Visual disturbances	Nearly always present Positive/negative: • Linear or zigzag • Scotoma • Fortification spectra	Unusual • Complicated visual phenomenon
Paresthesias	Common (5–60 min)	Common (seconds to minutes)
Altered consciousness	Usually responsive	Responsive during aura, altered responsiveness during complex partial seizure
Olfactory	Very uncommon	More common
Aphasia	Common	Common
Déjà vu	Rare	Common

Differential diagnosis and concomitant diagnosis of migraine and epilepsy: clinical and EEG features

Attacks in migraine and epilepsy can be divided into four phases: (i) the premonitory phase, which occurs hours or days before the attack; (ii) the aura, which comes immediately before the headache in migraine, and represents a simple partial seizure in epilepsy; (iii) the headache or seizure; and (iv) the postdrome. Most people do not experience all four phases in every attack. The similarity in terminology between migraine and epilepsy does not imply similarity in mechanisms.

Premonitory phase

Premonitory, or prodromal, phenomena occur in approximately 60% of migraineurs [59,60]. Features include constitutional, autonomic, psychologic (depression, euphoria, irritability, restlessness, mental slowness, hyperactivity, fatigue and drowsiness) and neurologic (photophobia, phonophobia and hyperosmia). In one study, the most common premonitory symptoms were feeling tired/weary (72%), difficulty concentrating (51%) and stiff neck (50%) [61]. Migraineurs who reported premonitory symptoms accurately predicted their full-blown headaches 72% of the time. Among patients who were almost certain that attacks would occur, 93% had attacks [61].

Premonitory symptoms have been reported in 6–47% of the epilepsy population, and include mood changes, malaise, nausea, headache and impaired concentration [62–65]. For epilepsy, it is important to distinguish between a prodrome, which implies a pre-ictal state, and an aura, which is the first part of the seizure. While the presence of a prodrome is less common in epilepsy than in migraine, studies have reported premonitory symptoms ranging from hours to a full day preceding a clinical seizure [62–65].

Aura

In migraine, the aura is a complex of focal neurologic symptoms that precedes or accompanies an attack [66]. About 20–30% of migraineurs have migraine with aura [67,68]. The same patient may have headache without aura, headache with aura, and aura without headache [69]. Most aura symptoms develop slowly over 5 to 20 minutes and usually last for less than 60 minutes. The aura almost always includes visual features [70], but somatosensory, motor, language and brainstem disturbances are not rare [69]. The mechanism of migraine aura is widely thought to be cortical spreading depression, a neuronal and glial event that includes both excitation and inhibition [29–32].

The visual aura of migraine often has a hemianoptic distribution and includes both positive (scintillations, fortification spectra, photopsia) and negative (scotoma) features. Elementary visual disturbances include colorless scotoma, photopsia or phosphenes. Simple flashes, specks or hallucinations of geometric forms (points, stars, lines, curves, circles, sparks, flashes or flames) occur and may be single or number in the hundreds. More complicated hallucinations include teichopsia, or fortification spectrum, which is the most characteristic visual aura and is almost diagnostic of migraine [67,69].

The aura in epilepsy is defined by the ILAE classification as 'that portion of the seizure which occurs before consciousness is lost, and for which memory is retained afterwards' [53]. The aura represents a simple partial non-motor seizure that typically precedes an observable seizure, but may occur alone. Auras are rapid in development, typically brief, and subjective only; in contrast to a complex partial or generalized seizure, they are not discernible to an outside observer [71]. Auras in epilepsy are often associated with symptoms that are unusual in migraine aura, frequently including autonomic or limbic sensations. Visual auras in epilepsy are infrequent; when present, they last for only seconds (with the rare exception of persistent visual auras), and are often associated with head or eye movement and subsequent alteration of consciousness [72]. The aura is associated with the electroencephalographic correlate of the seizure type in which it occurs; however, the EEG pattern is often not evident on surface recording until the seizure has progressed to involve a larger area of cortex.

Formed visual hallucinations are rare in migraine; when present in epilepsy, this manifestation may localize the seizure onset to the temporal or temporo-occipital region [72,73]. A comparison between auras of migraine and epilepsy is presented (see Tables 5.1 and 5.2).

Ictus (headache/seizure phase)

The typical migraine headache is unilateral and described as throbbing by 85% of patients. Headache severity ranges from moderate to marked and is aggravated by head movement or physical activity. The onset is usually gradual and the attack usually lasts 4 to 72 hours in adults and 2 to 48 hours in children. Anorexia is common, although food cravings can occur. Nausea occurs in up to 90% of patients, and vomiting occurs in about one-third of migraineurs. Many patients experience photophobia, phonophobia and osmophobia, and seek a dark, quiet room [74,75].

In contrast to the headache phase of migraine, the vast majority of seizures are self-limited and brief; it is estimated that over 90% of generalized tonic clonic seizures terminate within 2 minutes [76], although prolonged seizures (duration >5 and <30 minutes) and status epilepticus (duration ≥30 minutes) do occur. The clinical signs or symptoms of seizures depend on the region of the abnormal cortical discharges and the extent and pattern of the discharge propagation. A hallmark of the seizure phase of partial seizures, excluding simple partial seizures (which are the epileptic aura) is a change in the level of consciousness. Complex partial seizures are characterized by altered consciousness, while full loss of consciousness is present during generalized tonic clonic seizures [53]. Other features of complex partial seizures include automatisms (purposeless repetitive movements), vocalizations and posturing; features of generalized tonic clonic seizures include tonic clonic movements, incontinence and tongue biting.

Postdrome or post-ictal phase

With migraine, the patient may feel tired, washed out, irritable and listless and may have impaired concentration. Many patients report scalp tenderness. Some people feel unusually refreshed or euphoric after an attack, whereas others note depression and malaise. In epilepsy, during the post-ictal phase, there may be a depressed level of awareness or focal neurologic deficits [77] that sometimes provide clues to the site of seizure onset.

Seizure-associated headache

Headaches (not necessarily migraine) may occur before (pre-ictal), during (ictal) or after (post-ictal) a seizure [17]. Pre-ictal and ictal headaches are often neglected, because the seizure overshadows the headache for both patient and physician. Ictal headaches can occur with seizures as the sole or predominant clinical manifestation [78]. Isler et al. [79] found that hemicranial attacks of pain coincided with seizure activity and typically lasted seconds to minutes (hemicrania epileptica); in rare cases, ictal headache may last hours.

Electroencephalogram (EEG) in the diagnosis of migraine and epilepsy

While the EEG is extraordinarily useful in diagnosing epilepsy and differentiating subtypes, it is less valuable in diagnosing migraine. EEGs recorded during an attack of migraine with aura, unlike those recorded during a clinical seizure, are usually normal. Focal slowing sometimes occurs during migraine auras, although this is not a consistent finding. Previously recommended EEG markers of migraine, such as robust photic driving at high flash frequencies and slowing with hyperventilation, can be seen in children without a history of migraine and are not very specific [80]. Striking EEG patterns have been described in specific subtypes of migraine [81], such as paroxysmal lateralized epileptiform discharges (PLEDs) in association with hemiplegic migraine, prolonged migraine aura or incipient migrainous infarction.

The incidence of epileptiform activity in patients with migraine appears to be higher than that of the general population. However, this finding does not contribute to the diagnosis of patients with migraine, and may in fact confuse the issue [82]. EEG does not identify headache subtypes, or effectively screen for structural causes of headache, and is not useful in the routine assessment of headache patients [83]. The EEG is useful if headache patients have symptoms that suggest a seizure disorder, such as atypical migrainous aura or episodic loss of consciousness [80]. However, there is clearly a role for 24-hour closed-circuit television EEG recording when differentiating migraine aura from epileptic aura is difficult on clinical grounds, as illustrated by our patient history. It can also facilitate the diagnosis of comorbid epilepsy and migraine as well as the migralepsy syndrome [56].

Migraine variants commonly confused with epilepsy

Basilar-type migraine and confusional migraine

Basilar or basilar artery migraine is a variant of migraine with aura with at least one of the following aura features: ataxia, vertigo, tinnitus, diplopia, nystagmus, dysarthria, bilateral paresthesia, or a change in the levels of consciousness and cognition [84,85]. Confusional migraine is no longer part of the ICHD-2 classification. It is believed to represent a form of basilar-type migraine or hemiplegic migraine. During the confused period the patient is inattentive, distracted, and has difficulty maintaining speech and other motor activities. The EEG may be abnormal during the attack. A more profoundly disturbed level of consciousness may lead to migraine stupor, which can last from hours up to 5 days. The confusional state is usually followed by sleep, resembling post-ictal depression of mental status. Basilar migraine may be difficult to differentiate from simple or complex partial seizures or the post-ictal state following a primary or secondary generalized seizure [86].

Benign paroxysmal vertigo of childhood

This disorder is characterized by recurrent, brief episodic attacks of vertigo. It is now classified as one of the 'Childhood periodic syndromes' (ICHD-II 1.3.3) and is viewed as a precursor of migraine [87]. Attacks occur without warning and resolve spontaneously in otherwise healthy children. They last a few minutes and tend to recur at irregular intervals over a period of 6 to 12 months. Children with this disorder cannot stand, and lie silently on the floor or wish to be held during attacks. Although headache may not be present at the onset, as the disorder evolves the vertigo may be replaced by attacks of headache and vomiting, facilitating diagnosis. Vertigo as a manifestation of simple partial seizures is usually less prominent than in migraine.

Aura without headache

Migraine aura can occur without headache [88] although the diagnosis is more difficult in this setting and should be accepted as migraine only after a full investigation. Headache occurring in association with some attacks will help confirm the diagnosis. Late-life migrainous accompaniments are characterized by attacks of aura without headache beginning in late life [89,90]. Many patients have a history of migraine in early or midlife, often with an attack-free hiatus. Because focal neurologic defects occur without headache, they can be confused with TIAs or seizures [89,90].

Migraine-epilepsy syndromes

Migraine-triggered seizure

The association between migraine and epilepsy also occasionally occurs in a temporal relationship known as migralepsy. According to the ICHD-2 [6], migralepsy happens when seizures occur during or within one hour of a migraine aura. Rates of migralepsy reported in populations with comorbid migraine and epilepsy range from 1.7% to 16% [8,12]. Reported risk factors for migralepsy include attacks of migraine with aura and catamenial epilepsy [12]. In the case presented at the beginning of this chapter, the patient had a migraine aura and then developed a partial seizure with secondary generalization. This pattern is compatible with migralepsy.

Benign partial epilepsy of childhood with occipital paroxysms

Two occipital electroclinical syndromes, the early and late benign occipital epilepsies of childhood, often involve migraine-like symptoms and may represent a diagnostic challenge [91,92]. The early and more common form, also referred to as 'early onset benign childhood seizures with occipital spikes' (Panayiotopoulos syndrome), is a clinical syndrome consisting largely of autonomic seizures and autonomic status epilepticus [93]. Seizures comprise an unusual constellation of autonomic symptoms, mainly emetic symptoms of nausea, vomiting or retching, often with unilateral deviation of the eyes and other more conventional ictal manifestations. Other autonomic symptoms may occur, including pallor, flushing or cyanosis, mydriasis and, less often, miosis, coughing, cardiorespiratory and thermoregulatory alterations, incontinence of urine or feces, and gastrointestinal upset. Headache and, more often, cephalic auras that may be autonomic manifestations occur, particularly at onset. Confusion or loss of consciousness may ensue [91–93].

In contrast, the later onset form (Gastaut syndrome) is a less common clinical syndrome characterized by a partial seizure with visual symptoms, followed by post-ictal migraine and occipital spikes on EEG [94–96]. This syndrome has features of both epilepsy and migraine [94]. The visual symptoms may include amaurosis, elementary visual hallucinations (phosphenes), complex visual hallucinations, or visual illusions [97]. The visual symptoms are often followed by hemiclonic, complex partial, or secondarily generalized tonic-clonic seizures. Following the seizure, approximately 25–40% of the patients develop migraine-like headaches [96].

Benign rolandic epilepsy

Benign rolandic epilepsy, also referred to as benign epilepsy of childhood with centrotemporal spikes (BECT) and characterized by unilateral somatosensory or motor seizures and centrotemporal spikes, has been associated with migraine in some, but not all studies [98–101]. Speech arrest, pooling of saliva, and (usually) preservation of consciousness are typical, although secondary generalization may occur. The seizures almost invariably disappear by age 15. The association between benign rolandic epilepsy and migraine may be part of the comorbidity of migraine with all forms of epilepsy [99].

Treatment considerations

Because migraine and epilepsy are associated, clinicians should be sensitive to the issue of concomitant diagnoses. When diseases are comorbid, the principle of diagnostic parsimony does not apply. Individuals with one disorder are more likely, not less likely, to have the other. Epilepsy and migraine are fundamentally different disorders, mandating significant differences in approach to therapy. Nevertheless, many of the treatments for both disorders target the underlying neuronal hyperexcitability common to both [(22,102] thus allowing for overlap in treatment.

When planning treatment strategies for epilepsy and migraine, the possibility of comorbid disease should be considered [103]. Although tricyclic antidepressants and neuroleptic drugs are often used to treat migraine in patients with active comorbid epilepsy, they are best used in combination with an effective antiepileptic agent, as these medications may lower seizure thresholds. When selecting drugs for migraine prophylaxis, it is sometimes advantageous to treat comorbid conditions with a single agent; for example, anticonvulsants with efficacy for both migraine and epilepsy (divalproex sodium and topiramate) should be considered in patients with both disorders [104].

Treatment modalities: acute and preventive

Treatment modalities in epilepsy and migraine fall into two categories: acute therapies, administered in the immediate setting of an attack; and preventive therapies, administered interictally (typically daily) to prevent attacks. Similarities and differences in treatment choices for epilepsy and migraine reflect pathophysiologic differences and also potential underutilization of treatment.

There is only minimal overlap in acute therapy for the two disorders, seen mainly in the setting of prolonged ictus, either status epilepticus or status migrainosis, where intravenous valproate sodium may be utilized [105]. Benzodiazepines, the mainstay of acute therapy of seizures, are rarely used for migraine. Widely used acute agents in migraine include triptans, which have no known antiepileptic properties and may indeed lower seizure threshold [106], as well as non-steroidal anti-inflammatory drugs (NSAIDs) and analgesics.

Nearly every patient with epilepsy is maintained on preventive therapy; in contrast, preventive therapy for migraine should be considered in patients with more than 2 days of headache-related disability or more than 4 days of migraine per month. Estimates from the American Migraine Prevalence and Prevention Study suggest that 40% of migraine sufferers meet those criteria while only 13% of migraine sufferers receive preventive treatment [107].

There are currently two medications with US Food and Drug Administration (FDA) approval for preventive treatment in both epilepsy and migraine, divalproex sodium and topiramate. Divalproex sodium is an FDA-approved anticonvulsant for migraine prophylaxis. The efficacy of divalproex has been supported by open and double-blind, placebo-controlled studies [108–111]. The doses that are effective in migraine are generally lower than those used for epilepsy; 500 mg a day is often sufficient. Topiramate is a second FDA-approved anticonvulsant for migraine prophylaxis. In both open and placebo-controlled, double-blind trials, doses of 50 to 100 mg per day have been shown to be effective for migraine [112–114]. Other antiepileptic drugs that have been shown to be superior to placebo for migraine include gabapentin, levetiracetam, tiagabine, and zonisamide, but large-scale studies are needed. Lamotrigine may be effective for migraine aura, but not headache [115].

In addition, the recognition of potentially similar mechanisms and response to therapy between the disorders has led to crossover of other treatment modalities. For example, the Vagal Nerve Stimulator, an FDA-approved device for the add-on treatment of intractable partial epilepsy, is under investigation for migraine [116]. Similar efforts are likely to continue.

Clinical summary

In summary, migraine and epilepsy are comorbid conditions, and the presence of one disorder increases the likelihood of the other. Emerging data regarding shared genetics have begun to shed light on shared mechanisms of neuronal hyperexcitability. The comorbidity of migraine and epilepsy presents both pitfalls and opportunities, and the diagnosis and treatment of each disorder must take into account the potential presence of the other. Similarities in episode progression and symptoms may pose diagnostic challenges. The striking underlying mechanistic similarity in both disorders leads to therapeutic overlap, allowing each field to learn lessons from the other, in terms of both specific therapies and therapeutic strategies.

References

1 Andermann F. Migraine and epilepsy: an overview. In: Andermann F, Lugaresi E (eds) Migraine and epilepsy. Boston: Butterworths, 1987; 405–21.
2 Haut S, Bigal M, Lipton RBL. Chronic disorders with episodic manifestations: focus on epilepsy and migraine. Lancet Neurol 2006;5:148–57.
3 Andermann F. Clinical features of migraine-epilepsy syndrome. In: Andermann F, Lugaresi E (eds) Migraine and epilepsy. Boston: Butterworths, 1987; 3–30.
4 De Simone R, Ranieri A, Marano E, et al. Migraine and epilepsy: clinical and pathophysiological relations. Neurol Sci 2007;28(Suppl. 2): S150–5.
5 Silberstein SD, Saper JR, Freitag F. Migraine: diagnosis and treatment. In: Silberstein SD, Lipton RB, Dalessio DJ (eds) Wolff's Headache and Other Head Pain. New York: Oxford University Press, 2001; 121–237.
6 Headache Classification Committee. The International Classification of Headache Disorders, 2nd edn. Cephalalgia 2004;24(Suppl. 1):1–160.
7 Commission on Classification and Terminology of the International League Against Epilepsy. Proposal for revised classification of epilepsies and epileptic syndromes. Epilepsia 1989;30:389–99.
8 Marks DA, Ehrenberg BL. Migraine related seizures in adults with epilepsy, with EEG correlation. Neurology 1993;43:2476–83.
9 Andermann E, Andermann FA. Migraine-epilepsy relationships: epidemiological and genetic aspects. In: Andermann FA, Lugaresi E (eds) Migraine and Epilepsy. Boston: Butterworths, 1987; 281–91.
10 Ottman R, Lipton RB. Comorbidity of migraine and epilepsy. Neurology 1994;44:2105–10.
11 Lipton RB, Silberstein SD. Why study the comorbidity of migraine? Neurology 1994;44:4–5.
12 Velioglu SK, Ozmenoglu M. Migraine-related seizures in an epileptic population. Cephalalgia 1999;19:801.
13 Lipton RB, Ottman R, Ehrenberg BL, Hauser WA. Comorbidity of migraine: the connection between migraine and epilepsy. Neurology 1994;44 (Suppl. 7): 28–32.
14 Piccinelli P, Borgatti R, Nicoli F, et al. Relationship between migraine and epilepsy in pediatric age. Headache 2006:46:413–21
15 Ludvigsson P, Hesdorffer D, Olafsson E, Kjartansson O, Hauser WA. Migraine with aura is a risk factor for unprovoked seizures in children. Ann Neurol 2006;59:210–13.

16 Brodtkorb E, Bakken IJ, Sjaastad O. Comorbidity of migraine and epilepsy in a Norwegian community. Eur J Neurol 2008;15:1421–3.

17 Syvertsen M, Helde G, Stovner LJ, Brodtkorb EJ. Headaches add to the burden of epilepsy. Headache Pain 2007;8:224–30.

18 Solomon, S. Posttraumatic migraine, Headache 1998;38:772–8.

19 Frey LC. Epidemiology of posttraumatic epilepsy: a critical review. Epilepsia 2003;44(Suppl. 10):11–17.

20 Annegers JF, Rocca WA, Hauser WA. Causes of epilepsy: contributions of the Rochester epidemiology project. Mayo Clin Proc 1996;71:570–5.

21 Ottman R, Lipton RB. Is the comorbidity of epilepsy and migraine due to a shared genetic susceptibility? Neurology 1996;47:918–24.

22 Rogawski, M. Common pathophysiologic mechanisms of migraine and epilepsy. Arch Neurol 2008:65:709–14.

23 Roll P, Szepetowski P. Epilepsy and ionic channels. Epileptic Disord 2002;4:165–72.

24 Aroniadou-Anderjaska V, Fritsch B, Qashu F, Braga FM. Pathology and pathophysiology of the amygdala in epileptogenesis and epilepsy. J Epilep Res 2008;78:102–16.

25 Reid CA, Berkovic SF, Petrou S. Mechanisms of human inherited epilepsies. Prog Neurobiol 2009;87:41–57.

26 Moskowitz MA, Bolay H, Dalkara T. Migraine mechanisms: clues from familial hemiplegic migraine genotypes. Ann Neurol 2004;55:276–80.

27 Chang BSA, Lowenstein DH. Epilepsy. N Engl J Med 2003;349:1257–66.

28 Koch UR, Musshoff U, Pannek HW, et al. Intrinsic excitability, synaptic potentials, and short-term plasticity in human epileptic neocortex. J Neurosci Res 2005;80:715–26.

29 Aurora SK, Cao Y, Bowyer SM, Welch KM. The occipital cortex is hyperexcitable in migraine: experimental evidence. Headache 1999;39:469–76.

30 Olesen J, Larsen B, Lauritzen M. Focal hyperemia followed by spreading oligemia and impaired activation of RCBF in classic migraine. Ann Neurol 1981;9:344–52.

31 Lauritzen M. Pathophysiology of the migraine aura. The spreading depression theory. Brain 1994;117:199–210.

32 Olesen J, Friberg L, Skyhoj-Olsen T. Timing and topography of cerebral blood flow, aura and headache during migraine attacks. Ann Neurol 1990;28:791–8.

33 Vikelis M, Mitsikostas DD. The role of glutamate and its receptors in migraine. CNS Neurol Disord Drug Targets 2007;6:251–7.

34 Sanchez-Del-Rio M, Reuter U, Moskowitz MA. New insights into migraine pathophysiology. Curr Opin Neurol 2006;19:294–8.

35 Haan J, Terwindt GM, van den Maagdenberg AM, Stam AH, Ferrari MD. A review of the genetic relation between migraine and epilepsy, Cephalalgia 2008;28:105–11.

36 Joutel A, Bousser MG, Biousse V, et al. A gene for familial hemiplegic migraine maps to chromosome 19. Nat Genet 1993;5:40–5.

37 Ophoff RA, Terwindt GM, Vergouwe MN, et al. Familial hemiplegic migraine and episodic ataxia type-2 are caused by mutations in the Ca^{2+} channel gene CACNL1A4. Cell 1996;87:543–55.

38 Ophoff RA, van Eijk R, Sandkuijl LA, et al. Genetic heterogeneity of familial hemiplegic migraine. Genomics 1994;22:21–6.

39 Beauvais K, Cavé-Riant F, De Barace C, Tardieu M, Tournier-Lasserve E, Furby A. New CACNA1A gene mutation in a case of familial hemiplegic migraine with status epilepticus. Eur J Neurol 2004;52:58–61.

40 Kors EE, Melberg A, Vanmolkot KR, et al. Childhood epilepsy, familial hemiplegic migraine, cerebellar ataxia, and a new CACNA1A mutation. Neurology 2004;63:1136–7.

41 Tottene A, Fellin T, Pagnutti S, et al. Familial hemiplegic migraine mutations increase Ca^{2+} influx through single human CaV2.1 channels and decrease maximal CaV2.1 current density in neurons. Proc Natl Acad Sci USA 2002;99:13284–9.

42 Ducros A, Joutel A, Vahedi K, et al. Mapping of a second locus for familial hemiplegic migraine to 1q21-q23 and evidence of further heterogeneity. Ann Neurol 1997;42:885–90.

43 Gardner K, Barmada MM, Ptacek L, Hoffman E. A new locus for hemiplegic migraine maps to chromosome 1q31. Neurology 1997;49:1231–8.

44 Marconi R, De Fusco M, Aridon P, et al. Familial hemiplegic migraine type 2 is linked to 0.9Mb region on chromosome 1q23. Ann Neurol 2003;53:376–81.

45 De Fusco M, Marconi R, Silvestri L, et al. Haploinsufficiency of ATP1A2 encoding the Na^+/K^+ pump alpha-2 subunit associated with familial hemiplegic migraine type 2. Nat Genet 2003;33:192–6.

46 Vanmolkot KR, Kors EE, Hottenga JJ et al. Novel Mutations in the Na_,K_ -ATPase Pump Gene *ATP1A2* Associated with Familial Hemiplegic Migraine and Benign Female Infantile Convulsions. Ann Neurol 2003;54:360–6.

47 Lebas A, Guyant-Maréchal L, Hannequin D, Riant F, Tournier-Lasserve E, Parain D. Severe attacks of familial hemiplegic migraine, childhood epilepsy and ATP1A2 mutation. Cephalalgia 2008:28:774–7.

48 Dichgans M, Freilinger T, Eckstein G, et al. Mutation in the neuronal voltage-gated sodium channel SCN1A in familial hemiplegic migraine. Lancet 2005;366:371–7.

49 Escayg A, MacDonald BT, Meisler MH, et al. Mutations of SCN1A, encoding a neuronal sodium channel, in two families with GEFS+2. Nat Genet 2000;24:343–5.

50 Claes L, Del-Favero J, Ceulemans B, Lagae L, Van Broeckhoven C, De Jonghe P. De novo mutations in the sodium-channel gene SCN1A cause severe myoclonic epilepsy of infancy. Am J Hum Genet 2001;68:1327–32.

51 Ceulemans BP, Claes LR, Lagae LG. Clinical correlations of mutations in the SCN1A gene: from febrile seizures to severe myoclonic epilepsy in infancy Pediatr Neurol 2004;30:236–43.

52 Lossin C, Wang DW, Rhodes TH, Vanoye CG, George AL Jr. Molecular basis of an inherited epilepsy. Neuron 2002;34:877–84.

53 Commission on Classification and Terminology of the International League Against Epilepsy. Proposal for revised clinical and electrographic classification of epileptic seizures. Epilepsia 1981;22:489–501.

54 Hauser WA, Rich SS, Lee JR, Annegars JF, Anderson VE. Risk of recurrent seizures after two unprovoked seizures. N Engl J Med 1998;338:429–34.

55 Haut S. Differentiating migraine from epilepsy. Adv Std Med 2005;5(6E):S658–65.

56 Ehrenberg BL. Unusual clinical manifestations of migraine, and "the borderland of epilepsy" re-explored. Semin Neurol 1991;11:118–27.

57 So N. Epileptic auras. In: Wyllie E (ed.) The Treatment of Epilepsy: Principles and Practice, 3rd edn. Philadelphia: Lippincott Williams & Wilkins, 2001;229–239.

58 Hockaday JM. Equivalents of childhood migraine. In: Hockaday JM (ed.) Migraine in Childhood. Boston: Butterworths, 1988; 54–62.

59 Waelkens J. Warning symptoms in migraine: characteristics and therapeutic implications. Cephalalgia 1985;5:223–8.

60 Blau JN. Migraine prodromes separated from the aura: complete migraine. Br Med J 1980;281:658–60.

61 Giffin NJ, Ruggiero L, Lipton RB, et al. A novel approach to the study of premonitory symptoms in migraine using an electronic diary. Neurology 2003;60:935–40.

62 Hughes J, Devinsky O, Feldmann E, Bromfield E. Premonitory symptoms in epilepsy. Seizure 1993;2:201–3.

63 Rajna P, Clemens B, Csibri E, et al. Hungarian multicentre epidemiologic study of the warning and initial symptoms (prodrome, aura) of epileptic seizures. Seizure 1997;6:361–8.

64 Schulze-Bonhage A, Kurth C, Carius A, Steinhoff BJ, Mayer T. Seizure anticipation by patients with focal and generalized epilepsy: a multicentre assessment of premonitory symptoms. Epilepsy Res 2006;70:83–8.

65 Scaramelli A, Braga P, Avellanal A, et al. Prodromal symptoms in epileptic patients: clinical characterization of the pre-ictal phase. Seizure 2009,18;246–50.

66 Ziegler DK, Hassanein RS. Specific headache phenomena: their frequency and coincidence. Headache 1990;30:152–6.

67 Silberstein SD, Young WB. Migraine aura and prodrome. Semin Neurol 1995;45:175–82.

68 Walter F, Stewart WF, Linet MS, Celentano DD, Van Natta M, Ziegler D. Age- and sex-specific incidence rates of migraine with and without visual aura. Am J Epidemiol 1991;134:1111–20.

69 Russell M, Olesen J. A nosographic analysis of the migraine aura in a general population. Brain 1996;119:355–61.

70 Eriksen MK, Thomsen LL, Olesen J. The Visual Aura Rating Scale (VARS) for migraine aura diagnosis. Cephalalgia 2005;25:801–10.

71 Dreifuss R. Classification of epileptic seizures. In: Engel J, Pedley T (eds) Epilepsy: Comprehensive Textbook. Wolters Kluwer, 1999; 517–24.

72 Panayiotopoulos CP. Elementary visual hallucinations in migraine and epilepsy. J Neurol Neurosurg Psychiatry 1994;57:1371–4.

73 Bien CG, Benninger FO, Urbach H, Schramm J, Kurthen M, Elger CE. Localizing value of epileptic visual auras. Brain 2000;123:244–53.

74 Drummond PD. A quantitative assessment of photophobia in migraine and tension headache. Headache 1986;26:465–9.

75 Selby G, Lance JW. Observation on 500 cases of migraine and allied vascular headaches. J Neurol Neurosurg Psychiatry 1960;23:23–32.

76 Theodore WH, Porter JR, Albert P, et al. The secondarily generalized tonic-clonic seizure: a videotape analysis. Neurology 1994;44:1403–7.

77 Gallmetzer P, Leutmezer F, Serles W, Assem-Hilger E, Spatt J, Baumgartner C. Postictal paresis in focal epilepsies – incidence, duration, and causes: a video-EEG monitoring study. Neurology 2004;62:2160–4.

78 LaPlante P, Saint-Hilaire JM, Bouvier G. Headache as an epileptic manifestation. Neurology 1983;33:1493.

79 Isler H, Wirsen ML, Elli N. Hemicrania epileptica: synchronous ipsilateral ictal headache with migraine features. In: Andermann F, Lugaresi E (eds) Migraine and Epilepsy. Boston: Butterworths, 1987; 246–63.

80 Gronseth GS, Greenberg MK. The utility of the electroencephalogram in the evaluation of patients presenting with headache: a review of the literature. Neurology 1995;45:1263–7.

81 Beaumanoir A, Jekiel M. Electrographic observations during attacks of classical migraine. In: Andermann F, Lugaresi E (eds) Migraine and Epilepsy. Boston: Butterworths, 1987; 163–80.

82 Schachter SC, Ito M, Wannamaker BB, et al. Incidence of spikes and paroxysmal rhythmic events in overnight ambulatory computer-assisted EEGs of normal subjects: a multicenter study. J Clin Neurophysiol 1998;15:251–5.

83 American Academy of Neurology Quality Standards Subcommittee. Practice parameter: the electroencephalogram in the evaluation of headache (summary statement). Report of the Quality Standards Subcommittee. Neurology 1995;45:1411–13.

84 Bickerstaff ER. Migraine variants and complications. In: Blau JN (ed.) Migraine: Clinical and Research Aspects. Baltimore: Johns Hopkins University Press, 1987; 234–8.

85 Hosking G. Special forms: variants of migraine in childhood. In: Hockaday JM (ed.) Migraine in Childhood. Boston: Butterworths, 1988; 35–53.

86 Panayiotopoulos CP. Basilar migraine: a review. In: Panayiotopoulos CP (ed.) Benign childhood partial seizures and related epileptic syndromes. London: John Libbey, 1999; 303–8.

87 Lindskog U, Odkvist L, Noaksson L, Wallquist J. Benign paroxysmal vertigo in childhood: a long-term follow-up. Headache 1999;39:33–7.

88 Whitty CWM. Migraine without headache. Lancet 1967;ii:283–5.

89 Fisher CM. Late life migraine accompaniments as a cause of unexplained transient ischemic attacks. Can J Neurol Sci 1980;7:9–17.

90 Fisher CM. Late-life migraine accompaniments – further experience. Stroke 1986;17:1033–42.

91 Panayiotopoulos CP, Michael M, Sanders S, Valeta T, Koutroumanidis M. Benign childhood focal epilepsies: assessment of established and newly recognized syndromes. Brain 2008;131:2264–86.

92 Panayiotopoulos CP. Differentiating occipital epilepsies from migraine with aura, acephalgic migraine and basilar migraine. In: Panayiotopoulos CP (ed.) Benign Childhood Partial Seizures and Related Epileptic Syndromes. London: John Libbey, 1999; 281–302.

93 Panayiotopoulos CP. Benign childhood epilepsy with occipital paroxysms: a 15-year prospective study. Ann Neurol 1989;26:51–6.

94 Gastaut H. A new type of epilepsy: benign partial epilepsy of childhood with occipital spike-waves. Clin Electroencephalogr 1982;13:13–22.

95 Gastaut H. Benign epilepsy of childhood with occipital paroxysms. In: Roger J, Dravet C, Bureau M, Dreifuss FE, Wolf P (eds) Epileptic Syndromes in Infancy, Childhood, and Adolescence. London: John Libbey, Eurotext Ltd, 1985; 150–8.

96 Talwar D, Rask CA, Torres F. Clinical manifestations in children with occipital spike-wave paroxysms. Epilepsia 1992;33:667–74.

97 Newton R, Aicardi J. Clinical findings in children with occipital spike-wave complexes suppressed by eye-opening. Neurology 1983;33:1526–9.

98 Bladin PF. The association of benign rolandic epilepsy with migraine. In: Andermann F, Lugaresi E (eds) Migraine and Epilepsy. Boston: Butterworth, 1987; 145–52.

99 Wirrell EC, Hamiwka LD. Do children with benign rolandic epilepsy have a higher prevalence of migraine than those with other partial epilepsies or nonepilepsy controls? Epilepsia 2006;47:1674–81.

100 Bladin PF, Papworth G. "Chuckling and glugging" seizures at night – sylvian spike epilepsy. Proc Aus Assoc Neurol 1974;11:171–5.

101 Giroud M, Couillaut G, Arnould S, Dauvergne M, Dumas R, Nivelon JL. Epilepsy with Rolandic paroxysms and migraine; a nonfortuitous association. Results of a controlled study. Pediatrie 1989;44:659–64.

102 Welch KM. Contemporary concepts of migraine pathogenesis. Neurology 2003;61(8 Suppl. 4):S2–8.

103 Silberstein SD, Dodick D, Freitag F, et al. Pharmacological approaches to managing migraine and associated comorbidities – clinical considerations for monotherapy versus polytherapy. Headache 2007;47:585–99.

104 Silberstein SD, Lipton RB. Overview of the diagnosis and treatment of migraine. Neurology 1994;44(Suppl. 7):6–16.

105 Norton J. Use of intravenous valproate sodium in status migraine. Headache 2000;40:755–7.

106 Bigal ME, Lipton RB, Krymchantowski AV. The medical management of migraine. Am J Ther 2004;11:130–40.

107 Lipton RB, Bigal ME, Diamond M, Freitag F, Reed ML, Stewart WF. Migraine prevalence, disease burden, and the need for preventive therapy, Neurology 2007;68:343–9.

108 Jensen R, Brinck T, Olesen J. Sodium valproate has a prophylactic effect in migraine without aura. Neurology 1994;44:647–51.

109 Mathew NT. Valproate in the treatment of persistent chronic daily headache. Headache 1990;30:301.

110 Sianard-Gainko J, Lenaerts M, Bastings E, Schoenen. Sodium valproate in severe migraine and tension-type headache: clinical efficacy and correlations with blood levels. Cephalalgia 1993;13:252.

111 Sorensen KV. Valproate: a new drug in migraine prophylaxis. Acta Neurol Scand 1988;78:346–8.

112 Silberstein SD, Neto W, Schmitt J, Jacobs D, MIGR-001 Study Group. Topiramate in migraine prevention: results of a large controlled trial. Arch Neurol 2004;61:490–5.

113 Brandes JL, Saper JR, Diamond M, et al. for the MIGR-002 Study Group. Topiramate for migraine prevention: a randomized controlled trial. JAMA 2004;291:965–73.

114 Lewis D, Winner P, Saper J. Randomized, double-blind, placebo-controlled study to evaluate the efficacy and safety of topiramate for migraine prevention in pediatric subjects 12 to 17 years of age. Pediatrics 2009;123:924–34.

115 Steiner TJ, Findley LJ, Yuen AW. Lamotrigine versus placebo in the prophylaxis of migraine with and without aura. Cephalalgia 1997;17:109–12.

116 Mauskop A. Vagus nerve stimulation relieves chronic refractory migraine and cluster headaches. Cephalalgia 2005;25:82–6.

6 Migraine and Other Pain Disorders

Lars Jacob Stovner[1], Knut Hagen[1] and Rami Burstein[2]

[1] Norwegian National Headache Centre, Department of Neuroscience, Norwegian University of Science and Technology and St Olav's Hospital, Trondheim, Norway
[2] Department of Anesthesia and Critical Care, Beth Israel Deaconess Medical Center, Harvard Medical School, Boston, MA, USA

Case presentation

A 52-year-old female nurse assistant, working both day and night shifts, was referred to a neurologist because of frequent headaches and possible medication overuse. She had previously been told by her family physician that she had typical migraine. The attacks had started before the age of 10, and had become gradually worse after the birth of her third child. She had kept a headache diary for 6 months, showing that she had headaches for 15–20 days per month.

Previous history: At 38 she was referred to a psychologist for depression and anxiety. She got some help from psychotherapy, and used anti-depressants (selective serotonin reuptake inhibitors, SSRIs) for 7 months, but still had a tendency to become depressed. At the age of 47 she had been to a rheumatologist because over several years she had experienced increasing problems with low back pain, pain in both hips and migrating pain in several joints (fingers, toes, ankles and wrists). No indications of inflammatory arthritis were found. As she also had pain and tenderness in neck, arms, shoulder and buttocks a tentative diagnosis of fibromyalgia was made, and physical exercise was recommended, in addition to physical therapy. The bodily pain, particularly in the neck, interfered with her sleep. She found, however, that both physical exercise and manipulation of the neck could elicit headaches. For her joint pain, especially the shoulder, she used the non-steroidal anti-inflammatory drug (NSAID) diclophenac regularly for several months, which finally resulted in stomach pain, possibly due to gastritis. This drug was discontinued, and she later used mostly paracetamol for this pain.

Treatment of headache: For her headache attacks she always used a triptan. These were almost always quite effective, but during the last months she got muscle pain and stiffness after taking the drug. She had previously tried two types of antihypertensives as migraine prophylactics (propranolol and candesartan); the latter had seemingly been quite effective for half a year, but then the effect had tapered off. Once, her primary physician had

Comorbidity in Migraine, First Edition. Edited by J. Schoenen, D. W. Dodick and P. S. Sándor.
© 2011 Blackwell Publishing Ltd. Published 2011 by Blackwell Publishing Ltd.

also persuaded her to discontinue medication, but she got very much
worse during the five days without a triptan, and her shoulder pain
also became much worse, so she resumed medication, both triptans
and diclophenac, on day six. She had once declined to use a tricyclic
antidepressant (amitriptyline) for her headache because she had been
warned about side effects when she previously had been treated for
depression.

Comments: This is a very common patient in neurology practice and
specialized headache centers, demonstrating some of the complexities when
migraine and musculoskeletal pain occur in the same patient. In addition
to the 'primary' comorbidity, which may be constitutional due to common
pathophysiological mechanisms, this case also demonstrates that some of
the pain may occur as a complication of the treatment. For example, she got
muscle stiffness after taking triptans and stomach ache due to NSAIDs, and
physiotherapy for neck pain could elicit migraine attacks. In addition, the
shoulder pain was one reason why she did not manage to discontinue
analgesics in the attempt to treat her possible medication overuse headache.
Also, the neck pain interfered with her sleep, which might worsen her
migraines.

Probably, she should try once more to discontinue acute headache
medication, but this time she should be better prepared for the abstinence,
and she should be allowed to take some painkiller for her other pains. As
prophylactic medication, amitriptyline would be a logical choice because it
can be helpful for both migraine and fibromyalgia, and it may improve the
sleep quality and her depression. Starting at a low dose and increasing it
slowly would hopefully reduce side effects. It could be combined with other
migraine prophylactics like valproate or topiramate. A change in her job
should be considered as working night shifts may be particularly hard for a
migraine patient, for whom regular sleep is usually recommended. Active
physical therapy with advice on how to perform exercises and gradual
increase in physical activity may be helpful for patients with chronic
headache and fibromyalgia.

Introduction

Until now, a principal concern of headache science has been to analyze
and define the various headache disorders, with the aim of differentiating
between nosologically distinct subtypes that may be specific with regard
to pathogenetic mechanisms, genetic basis and treatment. This effort has
culminated in the International Classification of Headache Disorders
(ICHD) classification, with more than 200 different headache diagnoses
[1]. Compared to this great analytical endeavor there seems to have been
much less 'synthetic' scientific effort attempting to assess the degree of
relatedness between the different headache types, and between headaches
and other pain conditions. Defining what the headaches have in common

with other pain conditions, and what is unique to headache, may be important to gain a full understanding of these very prevalent and burdensome conditions, both for defining causes and risk factors and for finding the best treatment.

This chapter explores how headache is related to other pain disorders. To this purpose, all epidemiologic studies illuminating the degree to which headache conditions are comorbid with each other and with other pain conditions will be reviewed. In this regard, several mechanisms for comorbidities suggested by the epidemiologic evidence and also by clinical and experimental studies are discussed.

Comorbidity

In assessing whether two conditions are truly comorbid, in the sense that they co-occur in individuals more often than is expected by chance, several methodological fallacies must be eliminated. First, apparent comorbidity may exist if criteria for different disorders are overlapping. This is particularly important when comorbidity among different headache disorders is studied. Second, co-occurrence in clinical samples may be due to a so-called admission rate bias (Berkson's bias) since patients with two or more conditions are more likely to be admitted to hospitals or to seek a doctor. Third, associations between conditions should be controlled for confounding factors. In most studies, sex and age of individuals are controlled for, whereas adjustment for other important confounders such as socioeconomic status is often not done.

Epidemiologic evidence

Comorbidity between different headaches

Surprisingly few studies have investigated comorbidity between different headache disorders. One reason for this may be that criteria for the different headaches are partly overlapping, and therefore a careful history-taking by a headache specialist is necessary to make multiple valid diagnoses in the same individual. Such a procedure is expensive and time-consuming in population-based studies, and therefore only few such studies have been performed. In the 1989 Copenhagen study [2], the 1-year prevalence of tension-type headache (TTH) among migraineurs was 83% as compared with 73% among those without migraine ($p = 0.06$). In a later study of young adults [3], the corresponding figures were 94% and 85% [odds ratio (OR) 1.81; 95% confidence interval (CI) = 0.98–3.34], suggesting that there is a comorbidity between migraine and TTH. In a study from Norway [4], the lifetime prevalence of idiopathic stabbing headache was 35% among the general population, 38% among those with TTH and 45% among those with migraine with aura. As no confidence intervals are given, it is hard to evaluate whether the figures are coincidental. From a clinical perspective, it has been pointed out that migraine may be overlooked in patients with several headache types, as diagnosis may tend to focus on the most frequently occurring headache, which is usually TTH [5].

Comorbidity between headache and other pain disorders

Presumably, overlapping criteria should be less of a problem when this type of comorbidity is studied. For unknown reasons, however, most studies on comorbidity between headache and other pain conditions have been performed among children and adolescents. One possibility may be that clinicians find that headaches often occur in connection with other pains in this age group, which may lead to more research.

In Finland, among 1290 schoolchildren aged 8–9 years [6], those with migraine tended to have otalgia, shoulder/neck pain, back pain and abdominal pain more often than children with non-migrainous headache. In contrast, the prevalence of limb pain, throat pain, chest pain and toothache was similar among the two groups. This was contrary to the authors' expectation that non-migrainous headaches would be more associated with these other pains because they are considered to have a muscular origin. Children with migraine had more frequent headache attacks than children with non-migrainous headache. Among those with non-migrainous headache there was an association between attack frequency and non-headache pains, but not among the migraineurs. In the same country, among almost 2000 8-year-old children [7], there were statistically significant comorbidities between headache and abdominal (OR 2.3; 95% CI = 1.6–3.5) and other pain (OR 3.8; 95% CI = 2.7–5.8). In a cohort study of a Norwegian rural community that followed children between the ages of 4 and 10 [8], headache was rare at the youngest age (1.5%). Although no confidence intervals were given, abdominal pain and headache seemed to be comorbid at both ages, albeit most marked at the older age. In a case-control study from the same country [9] among patients referred to a pediatric department for recurrent abdominal pain ($n = 40$) and among matched controls from the population ($n = 82$), headache occurred more often among the patients than among the controls ($p = 0.03$). In a study of pain complaints among 793 Swedish adolescents [10], two-thirds of those with frequent headache also complained of frequent pain involving muscles, back, abdomen, ears and teeth. A study among 5474 German children aged 7–14 [11] found a clear-cut association between headache, back and stomach pain, the association being most evident for those with frequent headache. No analysis was done for migraine as compared to non-migrainous headache. A study among Scottish schoolchildren showed that the presence of headache at baseline was a risk factor for persistent musculoskeletal pain 1 and 4 years later [12]. A cross-sectional study among more than 9000 Danish adolescents on comorbidity of low back pain showed that headache occurred significantly more often among those with this condition, and the comorbidity was stronger with increasing duration of the back pain [13].

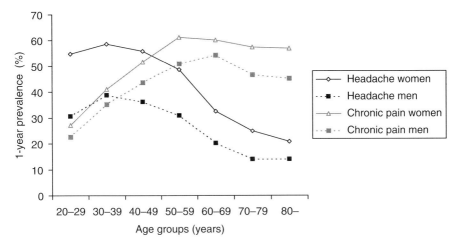

Figure 6.1 One-year prevalence of headache (n = 51,393) [54] and chronic musculoskeletal pain (*n* = 66,140) [55] in men and women, related to age, from the HUNT study.

Comparatively few studies exist for adults. In an adult population (20–84 years) of 8000 Swedes [14], headache was highly comorbid with shoulder pain, and painful conditions such as ulcer and dyspepsia. Using data from the 2002 National Health Interview survey in the USA [15], a population-based study among more than 30,000 adults indicated that self-reported severe headaches or migraine were more commonly associated with facial jaw pain (OR women 7.6, OR men 5.4), low back pain (OR 4.2 and 3.9) or neck pain (OR 6.6 and 2.5). In this study, adjustment was made for sociodemographic characteristics. From the same country, a population representative face-to-face survey among 5692 US adults [16] showed that chronic back pain, occurring in 19% of the population during the last year, was highly comorbid with both migraine (OR 5.2; 95% CI = 4.1–6.4) and other headaches (OR 4.0; 95% CI = 2.9–5.3).

Much information on the comorbidity of headache and other pains has come from the Norwegian HUNT studies. In these studies, comprising large numbers of health-related questionnaire data as well as biometric measurements of a large population (>50,000), the prevalence of chronic musculoskeletal pain (lasting ≥3 months) was almost twice as high among those with either migraine or non-migrainous headache compared to the general population [17]. Headache and chronic musculoskeletal pain were quite different with regard to the age distribution since the peak prevalence of headache was reached in the 40s, whereafter it tapered off, whereas musculoskeletal pain increased gradually until the 60s, but after this age the prevalence was relatively stable (Figure 6.1). There was no marked difference between those with migraine and non-migrainous headaches, but in all age groups, those with migraine or other headaches had a 15–20% higher prevalence of chronic musculoskeletal pain than those without headache, and there was a clear relation between frequency of headache and prevalence of musculoskeletal pain. Among those with

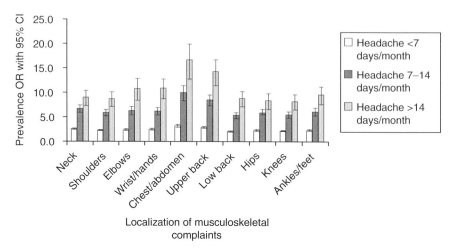

Figure 6.2 One-year prevalence of different headache frequency categories (<7 days/month, 7–14 days/month, and >14 days/month) related to 10 different localizations of musculoskeletal symptoms [odds ratios (ORs) with 95% confidence intervals (CI)]. Reference category (OR = 1.0): individuals without musculoskeletal symptoms. *n* = 47 557. Reproduced from Hagen et al. [17], with permission from Blackwell Publishing.

chronic headache (i.e. occurring more than 14 days per month) chronic musculoskeletal complaints were more than four times more prevalent than among those without headache. This was also the case for pain in areas far from the head, such as the ankle or knee (Figure 6.2). On the other hand, in those with pain restricted to one body area, neck pain was more closely related to headache than pain in other parts of the body.

Possible mechanisms for comorbidity of the pain disorders

If the observed comorbidities between the headaches and the different pain conditions are real, i.e. not due to confounding or bias, there are at least three theories to explain such comorbidity: (i) headache triggered by musculoskeletal pain; (ii) musculoskeletal pain triggered by headache; and (iii) underlying pathology or disposition that is common to both headache and musculoskeletal pain. It should be emphasized that an explanation of the observed comorbidity may involve all three mechanisms.

According to the first (the 'peripheral triggering theory'), musculoskeletal pains that originate in the neck, shoulder or jaw are capable of triggering headache. According to the second (the 'central convergence theory'), headache induces altered excitability in central trigeminovascular neurons that process nociceptive information from muscles of the neck and shoulders, as well as the jaws. In the past 30 years, a large number of studies have carefully documented the specifics of muscle tenderness that develops *before* the onset of headache [18–24].

Although a neural mechanism is lacking for the theory that muscle tenderness (or pains that originate in any extracranial organ) can trigger a headache, one cannot dismiss this option. In the past, attempts to provide a mechanistic explanation focused on activation of central trigeminovascular neurons by abnormal nociceptive input from muscles of the head, neck and shoulders. The concept of cervicogenic headache, believed to be a secondary headache stemming from pain in some neck structure, hinges on this concept [25]. This somewhat controversial entity may be fairly common [26]. However, the difficulty with this explanation is the scarcity of clinical evidence for skin, muscles and bone pains that may be referred to internal organs or trigger the perception of pain in visceral tissue. Most commonly, it is visceral pain that ends up being referred to external tissues such as muscles or skin. Preserving the viability of the peripheral theory is the possibility that pain signals that originate in tender muscles and facial joints, trigger a migraine-type headache involving activation of intracranial pain fibers, through a connection that is not yet understood.

Another reasonable way to explain headache comorbidity with chronic musculoskeletal pain is the central convergence theory (Figure 6.3). According to this theory, the spinal trigeminal nucleus contains second-order lamina V neurons that receive sensory information from the meninges, pericranial and neck muscles, facial skin, upper teeth and temporomandibular joint [27,28]. If activated for a long period of time during repeated headache attacks, these neurons can undergo molecular changes that alter the physiologic properties of their membrane and render them hyperexcitable and sensitized [28]. When sensitized, these neurons tend to process non-painful sensory signals that originate in muscles, skin and joints as if they were painful [29,30]. This results in the perception of muscle tenderness, joint pain and cutaneous allodynia. Whereas this scenario can explain comorbidity between different headache types and between headache and musculoskeletal pain in the neck, shoulders and pericranial muscles, it falls short of explaining how headache can be comorbid with, for example, abdominal and low-back pain. Adhering to the same principle, it may be that sensitization of neurons that are activated during a headache and process sensory information from muscles innervated by lumbosacral dorsal root ganglia, can elucidate headache comorbidity with low back pain. Such neurons are found in the thalamus [31] and caudal ventrolateral medulla [32].

A general hyperexcitability could also develop along nociceptive dorsal horn neurons in the spinal cord following the activation of descending pathways that facilitate pain processing [33,34] or the suppression of descending pathways that slow pain transmission [35]. Repeated migraine attacks are thought to produce cumulative adverse effects on the function of brainstem regions that modulate pain processing [36]. Recent imaging studies showing abnormal periaqueductal gray matter (PAG) activation during migraine [37] and deposition of abnormally high levels of iron in patients with a long history of migraine [36], have helped this theory gain momentum. Since the threshold for activation of nociceptive dorsal horn

Theory of central convergence

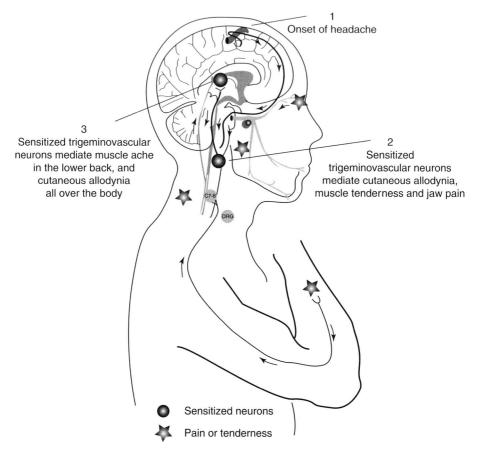

Figure 6.3 Theory of central convergence. Second-order neurons in the spinal trigeminal nucleus are activated and sensitized following repeated excitation during headache. Ongoing activity that develops in spinal trigeminal nucleus neurons is later relayed to third-order neurons in the thalamus and sensitizes them. Sensitization of spinal and thalamic neurons can mediate musculoskeletal and joint pain from neck, shoulders and lower back, respectively. DRG: dorsal root ganglion.

neurons depends on the balance between incoming nociceptive signals from the periphery and their modulation by spinal and supraspinal pathways, any change in modulation can render the spinal cord neurons hyperexcitable; the consequence of this is their activation by subthreshold stimuli (excitatory postsynaptic potentials) or by non-noxious stimuli such as mild stretching of a muscle.

The third explanation for the comorbidity is that patients with different pain disorders share some common underlying factor or disposition related to pain processing. Recent years have seen some interesting epidemiologic evidence supporting this hypothesis. In the HUNT studies referred to above, showing comorbidity between headache and other pain

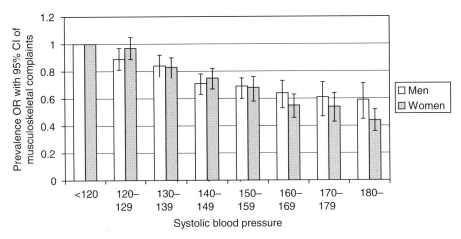

Figure 6.4 One-year prevalence of chronic musculoskeletal pain related to systolic blood pressure level among 66,140 men and women (from the HUNT study [40]).

conditions, the prevalence of headache (migraine and non-migrainous headache) [38,39] as well as pain in all other body regions, was inversely related to blood pressure, among both men and women. For chronic musculoskeletal pain, this was demonstrated both for the systolic (Figure 6.4) and the diastolic blood pressure [40]. For headache and migraine, the association was most conspicuous for the pulse pressure (difference between the systolic and diastolic blood pressure; Figure 6.5) [39]. This was the case in the cross-sectional study where blood pressure and pain were registered during the same period, and in the prospective design where blood pressure was registered 11 years earlier. This inverse relation was present for all age groups, both for headache and for chronic musculoskeletal pain.

The inverse association between pain and blood pressure has also been made by other groups. A Brazilian study concluded that migraine was more prevalent among those with optimal blood pressure than among those with hypertension [41]. A French study gave similar results and also demonstrated that migraine was inversely related to carotid wall thickness, indicating a lower sensitivity of the baroreceptors [42]. An Icelandic study showed that migraineurs tended to have lower systolic but higher diastolic pressures than non-migraineurs [43]. Much less evidence exists for other pains, but it has been found that hypertensive patients experience less intense pain during angina and myocardial infarction than normotensive patients [44].

The most likely explanation for this finding is hypertension-related hypalgesia. This phenomenon was first observed in rats, and it has subsequently been described in various animal and human pain models. A 1979 study [45] reported that increasing the blood pressure pharmacologically in rats reduced their avoidance reaction following a mildly aversive trigeminal nucleus stimulus. This effect was not seen in

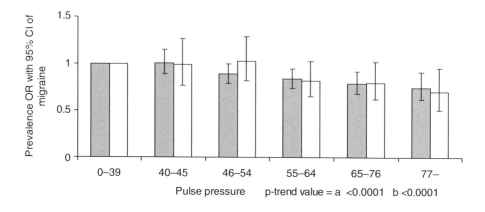

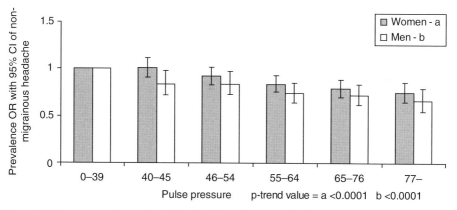

Figure 6.5 One-year prevalence of headache related to pulse pressure level in 51,130 men and women, from the HUNT study. Reproduced from Tronvik et al. [39] with permission from Lippincot, Williams & Wilkins.

rats with denervated baroreceptors. Since then, many studies have shown a diminished perception of painful stimuli in hypertensive individuals, independent of the method used to increase blood pressure (by pharmacological means, increasing salt intake, or with surgery to arteries) or to deliver nociceptive stimuli [46]. Spinal transmission of nociceptive stimuli is diminished in spontaneously hypertensive rats compared to normotensive rats [47], and hypertensive humans [48] have been shown to have decreased pain sensitivity to dental pulp stimulation. There is evidence that stimulation of the baroreflex arch due to increased blood pressure may inhibit pain transmission at both spinal and supraspinal levels, possibly due to interactions with brain areas that modulate nociception and cardiovascular reflexes in the brainstem [49]. This phenomenon is also present within the normotensive range, and the pain threshold is more closely associated with 24-hour arterial blood pressure than blood pressure values obtained just prior to induction of pain [50]. Anatomically, baroreceptors are well positioned to influence the activity of neurons in the nucleus tractus solitarius, locus caeruleus, paraventricular hypothalamus, paratrigeminal nucleus, PAG [51] and nucleus raphe magnus [45]. In humans we know that increased pulse pressure in healthy middle-aged subjects is associated with reduced baroreflex sensitivity [52], and a reduced baroreflex sensitivity has been shown to correlate with hypalgesia [53]. Whether hypertension-related hypalgesia is secondary to elevated blood pressure or whether they share some common mechanism is not yet known.

According to the HUNT studies, the effect of hypertension-associated hypalgesia on the prevalence of pain in the population is large: the prevalence of chronic musculoskeletal pain was 30–40% lower in those with systolic blood pressure (SBP) above 160 mmHg compared to those with values below 160 mmHg, independently of pain localization, age, sex and occupation [40]. The headache prevalence was 20–30% lower in those with SBP above 150 mmHg compared to those with SBP below 140 mmHg [38]. If the blood pressure in some way reflects or even sets the general level of pain sensitivity, as the literature indicates, the HUNT data suggest that the general level of pain sensitivity is important in explaining the occurrence of pain conditions in the populations at large, and for explaining the comorbidity between headache and other pain conditions.

Diagnosing and handling patients with migraine and other pain conditions

It is important to know that one patient may have two or more primary headaches, or a primary and a secondary headache. In the very common situation in which a patient has both migraine and tension-type headache, each type should be diagnosed and treated optimally. Although rare, a patient with a primary headache may also develop a secondary headache. The ICHD-2 criteria require that for making a diagnosis of migraine or another primary headache, other possible causes should be ruled out. This is a precaution against attributing all pains in the head to, for example, the patient's migraine, with the risk that a dangerous or treatable secondary headache is overlooked. Therefore, potential 'local' causes of head pain should be considered and investigated with appropriate methods. On the other hand, it is important to understand that pains in areas adjacent to the head (face, neck, shoulders, etc.) may be components of a migraine or another primary headache. Too often headache is attributed to a dubious chronic sinusitis or dental condition, or to tender neck muscles, only because the pain may be felt in these areas or because of non-specific findings on supplementary investigations (e.g. neck, dental or sinus X-rays).

Handling a patient with both migraine and other pain, which is often widespread in the musculoskeletal system, may be a challenging task, and no therapeutic studies have specifically addressed patients with this comorbidity. Several of the problems in the management of these patients were discussed in the case at the start of the chapter. For the doctor it may be useful to realize from the start that an optimal treatment and rehabilitation of the patient may require that all pains are tended to. A thorough investigation for specific disorders (inflammatory arthritis, osteoarthrosis, disk herniations, polymyalgia rheumatica/temporal arteritis, etc.) may be indicated. It is often an advantage to have a multidisciplinary approach; for instance, it may be necessary to work with psychological tensions or family conflicts, improve the general physical fitness of the patient, or change poor ergonomic or other unfavorable working conditions. Since the most severely affected headache patients are those most likely to have comorbid musculoskeletal pain, medication overuse may often complicate the condition. The patient's use of medicines should be critically appraised, and the fact that some acute headache medicines can give rise to painful side effects or worsen headache if overused should be carefully explained to the patient. The common migraine prophylactic drugs (beta-blockers, candesartan, valproate, topiramate) may be effective, and in patients with prominent musculoskeletal pain the tricyclic antidepressants (e.g. amitriptyline) can be particularly helpful because they have a documented effect on not only migraine but also chronic tension-type headache and chronic widespread pain, and they may also restore sleep and relieve depression. Physical activity may be effective for both chronic headache and musculoskeletal pain, and physical exercise has the added advantage that it makes the patient an active participant in the treatment. Well-conducted studies on treatment of patients with such comorbidity, including instruments to register effect on all pain conditions, should have high priority.

Conclusion

The epidemiologic evidence has shown that migraine and other headaches are comorbid with other pain conditions in both sexes and all age groups. Although it is possible that pain from peripheral organs in the vicinity of the head can induce headache through sensitization of brainstem neurons, there is much more evidence for the opposite theory, that headache leads to pain in anatomical sites near the head through a neural mechanism of referred pain and central sensitization. Some observations also indicate that repeated migraine attacks may influence general pain-modulating systems in the brainstem, thereby explaining observed comorbidity between migraine and pain in parts of the body that are remote from the head. Such comorbidity may also be related to some other factors that lead to a general increase in pain sensitivity in some individuals; this gains support from the fact that the phenomenon of hypertension-associated hypalgesia seems to be as important for the headaches as for pain in all parts of the body. Gaining a better understanding of the neural substrate of comorbidity may shed much light on the pathophysiology of headache. Taking this comorbidity into consideration may also improve clinical outcome.

References

1 Headache Classification Subcommittee of the International Headache Society. The International Classification of Headache Disorders, 2nd edn. 2004.

2 Rasmussen BK, Jensen R, Schroll M, Olesen J. Epidemiology of headache in a general population – a prevalence study. J Clin Epidemiol 1991;44:1147–57.

3 Lyngberg AC, Rasmussen BK, Jorgensen T, Jensen R. Has the prevalence of migraine and tension-type headache changed over a 12-year period? A Danish population survey. Eur J Epidemiol 2005;20:243–9.

4 Sjaastad O, Pettersen H, Bakketeig LS. The Vaga study; epidemiology of headache I: the prevalence of ultrashort paroxysms. Cephalalgia 2001;21:207–15.

5 Diamond ML. The role of concomitant headache types and non-headache co-morbidities in the underdiagnosis of migraine. Neurology 2002;58(9 Suppl. 6):S3–S9.

6 Anttila P, Metsahonkala L, Mikkelsson M, Helenius H, Sillanpaa M. Comorbidity of other pains in schoolchildren with migraine or nonmigrainous headache. J Pediatr 2001;138:176–80.

7 Santalahti P, Aromaa M, Sourander A, Helenius H, Piha J. Have there been changes in children's psychosomatic symptoms? A 10-year comparison from Finland. Pediatrics 2005;115:e434–e42.

8 Borge AI, Nordhagen R, Moe B, Botten G, Bakketeig LS. Prevalence and persistence of stomach ache and headache among children. Follow-up of a cohort of Norwegian children from 4 to 10 years of age. Acta Paediatr 1994;83:433–7.

9 Stordal K, Nygaard EA, Bentsen BS. Recurrent abdominal pain: a five-year follow-up study. Acta Paediatr 2005;94:234–6.

10 Fichtel A, Larsson B. Psychosocial impact of headache and comorbidity with other pains among Swedish school adolescents. Headache 2002;42:766–75.

11 Kroner-Herwig B, Heinrich M, Morris L. Headache in German children and adolescents: a population-based epidemiological study. Cephalalgia 2007;27:519–27.

12 El-Metwally A, Halder S, Thompson D, Macfarlane GJ, Jones GT. Predictors of abdominal pain in schoolchildren: a 4-year population-based prospective study. Arch Dis Child 2007;92:1094–8.

13 Hestbaek L, Leboeuf-Yde C, Kyvik KO, et al. Comorbidity with low back pain: a cross-sectional population-based survey of 12- to 22-year-olds. Spine 2004;29:1483–91; discussion 92.

14 Bingefors K, Isacson D. Epidemiology, co-morbidity, and impact on health-related quality of life of self-reported headache and musculoskeletal pain – a gender perspective. Eur J Pain 2004;8:435–50.

15 Strine TW, Chapman DP, Balluz LS. Population-based U.S. study of severe headaches in adults: psychological distress and comorbidities. Headache 2006;46:223–32.

16 Von Korff M, Crane P, Lane M, et al. Chronic spinal pain and physical-mental comorbidity in the United States: results from the national comorbidity survey replication. Pain 2005;113:331–9.

17 Hagen K, Einarsen C, Zwart JA, Svebak S, Bovim G. The co-occurrence of headache and musculoskeletal symptoms amongst 51 050 adults in Norway. Eur J Neurol 2002;9:527–33.

18 Ashina M, Bendtsen L, Jensen R, Sakai F, Olesen J. Muscle hardness in patients with chronic tension-type headache: relation to actual headache state. Pain 1999;79:201–5.

19 Ashina S, Jensen R, Bendtsen L. Pain sensitivity in pericranial and extracranial regions. Cephalalgia 2003;23:456–62.

20 Tfelt-Hansen P, Lous I, Olesen J. Prevalence and significance of muscle tenderness during common migraine attacks. Headache 1981;21:49–54.

21 Lous I, Olesen J. Evaluation of pericranial tenderness and oral function in patients with common migraine, muscle contraction headache and 'combination headache'. Pain 1982;12:385–93.

22 Jensen K, Tuxen C, Olesen J. Pericranial muscle tenderness and pressure-pain threshold in the temporal region during common migraine. Pain 1988;35:65–70.

23 Jensen R, Rasmussen BK, Pedersen B, Lous I, Olesen J. Prevalence of oromandibular dysfunction in a general population. J Orofacial Pain 1993;7:175–82.

24 Jensen K. Extracranial blood flow, pain and tenderness in migraine. Clinical and experimental studies. Acta Neurol Scand Suppl 1993;147:1–27.

25 Göbel H, Edmeads JG. Disorders of the skull and cervical spine. In: Olesen J, Goadsby PJ, Ramadan NM, Tfelt-Hansen P, Welch KMA (eds) The Headaches, 3rd edn. Philadelphia: Lippincott Williams & Wilkins, 2006; 1003–11.

26 Sjaastad O, Bakketeig LS. Prevalence of cervicogenic headache: Vaga study of headache epidemiology. Acta Neurol Scand 2008;117:173–80.

27 Burstein R. Deconstructing migraine headache into peripheral and central sensitization. Pain 2001;89:107–10.

28 Burstein R, Levy D, Jakubowski M, Woolf CJ. Peripheral and central sensitization related to headache. In: Olesen J, Welch KMA, Goadsby PJ, Tfelt-Hansen P (eds) The Headaches. Philadelphia: Lippincott Williams & Wilkins, 2006; 119–26.

29 Burstein R, Yamamura H, Malick A, Strassman AM. Chemical stimulation of the intracranial dura induces enhanced responses to facial stimulation in brain stem trigeminal neurons. J Neurophysiol 1998;79:964–82.

30 Burstein R, Yarnitsky D, Goor-Aryeh I, Ransil BJ, Bajwa ZH. An association between migraine and cutaneous allodynia. Ann Neurol 2000;47:614–24.

31 Garcia-Nicas E, Jakubowski M, Burstein R. Sensitization of thalamic trigeminovascular neurons in VPM and PO by chemical stimulation of the dura: implication for extracranial allodynia during migraine. Society for Neuroscience Abstracts 2004;746:3.

32 Malick A, Strassman RM, Burstein R. Trigeminohypothalamic and reticulohypothalamic tract neurons in the upper cervical spinal cord and caudal medulla of the rat. J Neurophysiol 2000;84:2078–112.

33 Kovelowski CJ, Ossipov MH, Sun H, Lai J, Malan TP, Porreca F. Supraspinal cholecystokinin may drive tonic descending facilitation mechanisms to maintain neuropathic pain in the rat. Pain 2000;87:265–73.

34 Ossipov MH, Hong Sun T, Malan P Jr, Lai J, Porreca F. Mediation of spinal nerve injury induced tactile allodynia by descending facilitatory pathways in the dorsolateral funiculus in rats. Neurosci Lett 2000;290:129–32.

35 Fields HL, Basbaum AI. Central nervous system mechanisms of pain modulation. In: Wall PD, Melzack R (eds) Textbook of Pain. London: Churchill Livingstone, 1999; 243–57.

36 Welch KM, Nagesh V, Aurora SK, Gelman N. Periaqueductal gray matter dysfunction in migraine: cause or the burden of illness? Headache 2001;41:629–37.

37 Weiller C, May A, Limmroth V, et al. Brain stem activation in spontaneous human migraine attacks. Nat Med 1995;1:658–60.

38 Hagen K, Stovner LJ, Vatten L, Holmen J, Zwart JA, Bovim G. Blood pressure and risk of headache: a prospective study of 22685 adults in Norway. J Neurol Neurosurg Psychiatry 2002;72:463–6.

39 Tronvik E, Stovner LJ, Hagen K, Holmen J, Zwart JA. High pulse pressure protects against headache: prospective and cross-sectional data (HUNT study). Neurology 2008;70:1329–36.

40 Hagen K, Zwart JA, Holmen J, Svebak S, Bovim G, Stovner LJ. Does hypertension protect against chronic musculoskeletal complaints? The Nord-Trondelag Health Study. Arch Intern Med 2005;165:916–22.

41 Wiehe M, Fuchs SC, Moreira LB, Moraes RS, Fuchs FD. Migraine is more frequent in individuals with optimal and normal blood pressure: a population-based study. J Hypertens 2002;20:1303–6.

42 Tzourio C, Gagniere B, El Amrani M, Alperovitch A, Bousser MG. Relationship between migraine, blood pressure and carotid thickness. A population-based study in the elderly. Cephalalgia 2003;23:914–20.

43 Gudmundsson LS, Thorgeirsson G, Sigfusson N, Sigvaldason H, Johannsson M. Migraine patients have lower systolic but higher diastolic blood pressure compared with controls in a population-based study of 21,537 subjects. The Reykjavik Study. Cephalalgia 2006;26:436–44.

44 Falcone C, Auguadro C, Sconocchia R, Angoli L. Susceptibility to pain in hypertensive and normotensive patients with coronary artery disease: response to dental pulp stimulation. Hypertension 1997;30:1279–83.

45 Dworkin BR, Filewich RJ, Miller NE, Craigmyle N, Pickering TG. Baroreceptor activation reduces reactivity to noxious stimulation: implications for hypertension. Science 1979;205:1299–301.

46 Guasti L, Grimoldi P, Diolisi A, et al. Treatment with enalapril modifies the pain perception pattern in hypertensive patients. Hypertension 1998;31:1146–50.

47 Randich A, Robertson JD. Spinal nociceptive transmission in the spontaneously hypertensive and Wistar–Kyoto normotensive rat. Pain 1994;58:169–83.

48 Zamir N, Shuber E. Altered pain perception in hypertensive humans. Brain Res 1980;201:471–4.

49 Ghione S. Hypertension-associated hypalgesia. Evidence in experimental animals and humans, pathophysiological mechanisms, and potential clinical consequences. Hypertension 1996;28:494–504.

50 Guasti L, Cattaneo R, Rinaldi O, et al. Twenty-four-hour noninvasive blood pressure monitoring and pain perception. Hypertension 1995;25:1301–5.

51 Murphy AZ, Ennis M, Rizvi TA, Behbehani MM, Shipley MT. Fos expression induced by changes in arterial pressure is localized in distinct, longitudinally organized columns of neurons in the rat midbrain periaqueductal gray. J Comp Neurol 1995;360:286–300.

52 Virtanen R, Jula A, Huikuri H, et al. Increased pulse pressure is associated with reduced baroreflex sensitivity. J Hum Hypertens 2004;18:247–52.

53 Guasti L, Zanotta D, Mainardi LT, et al. Hypertension-related hypoalgesia, autonomic function and spontaneous baroreflex sensitivity. Auton Neurosci 2002;99:127–33.

54 Hagen K, Zwart JA, Vatten L, Stovner LJ, Bovim G. Prevalence of migraine and non-migrainous headache – head-HUNT, a large population-based study. Cephalalgia 2000;20:900–6.

55 Svebak S, Hagen K, Zwart J-A. One-year prevalence of chronic musculoskeletal pain in a large adult Norwegian county population: Relation with age and gender– the HUNT study. J Musculoskeletal Pain 2006;14:21–8.

7 Migraine and Medication Overuse

Stephen D. Silberstein

Jefferson Headache Center, Thomas Jefferson University Hospital, Philadelphia, PA 19107, USA

Introduction

Patients with frequent headaches often overuse analgesics, opioids, ergotamine and triptans [1]. Overuse may result in increasing headache frequency [2]. Anxiety, depression and other psychological disturbances frequently accompany headaches associated with medication overuse – medication overuse headache (MOH) [3]. MOH may be refractory to preventive medication [4–9]. It was first observed in Switzerland, where workers in the pharmaceutical industry were given free samples of phenacetin-containing pain medication at the workplace [10]. Peters and Horton [11] observed the same phenomenon in patients who used large amounts of ergotamine preparations; they described 52 patients who took ergotamine on a daily basis, developed daily headache, and significantly improved after ergotamine was withdrawn [12–14]. The triptans not only lead to MOH, but also may cause increased migraine frequency [15,16].

Although stopping the overused acute medication may result in withdrawal symptoms and a period of increased headache, subsequent headache improvement frequently occurs [2,9,17–19]. MOH patients who were withdrawn from ergotamine and analgesics and given no further therapy no longer had daily headaches, although about 40% still had episodic migraine attacks [20,21]. Many terms have been used to describe MOH, including rebound headache, medication-misuse headache, and drug-induced headache. In order to emphasize the *regular* intake of drugs as the basis of this headache form, the new International Headache Society (IHS) classification [22] uses the term MOH (Table 7.1).

It was formerly believed that MOH occurred if drug use exceeded 2 to 3 days a week, week after week, month after month [23], emphasizing frequency and reliability of use. According to the International Classification of Headache Disorders, 2nd Edition (ICHD-2), overuse is now defined in terms of treatment days per month and emphasizes frequency and regularity of days per week. For example, the diagnostic criterion of use on 10 or more days a month (15 for simple analgesics) translates into

---

Table 7.1 New International Headache Society (IHS) criteria for headache attributed to medication overuse.

A. Headache present on >15 days/month
B. Regular overuse for >3 months of one or more acute/symptomatic treatment drugs as defined under sub forms of 8.2.
    1. Ergotamine, triptans, opioids, **or** combination analgesic medications on ≥10 days/month on a regular basis for >3 months
    2. Simple analgesics **or** any combination of ergotamine, triptans, analgesic opioids on ≥15 days/month on a regular basis for >3 months without overuse of any single class alone
C. Headache has developed or markedly worsened during medication overuse

Adapted from Headache Classification Committee of the International Headache Society [92].

2 to 3 treatment days every week. Bunching treatment days and going for long periods without medication intake, as practiced by some patients, is much less likely to cause MOH. The amount of use that constitutes overuse depends on the drug. Ergotamine-, triptan-, opioid- or combination analgesic-overuse headache requires intake on 10 or more days a month on a regular basis for 3 or more months. This may occur sooner with triptan than with ergotamine overuse [24,25].

Epidemiology

Analgesics are widely overused. In a representative sample of the Swiss population, 4.4% of men and 6.8% of women took analgesics at least once a week, and 2.3% took them daily [26]. Swiss psychiatric inpatients had more frequent analgesic dependency than dependency on tranquilizers, hypnotics and stimulating drugs [27]. In Germany, 1% of the population may take up to 10 pain tablets every day [28]. In a cross-sectional survey carried out in Tromsø in 1986–87, 19,137 men and women (aged 12 to 56 years) from the general population were asked about their drug use over the preceding 14 days. On average, 28% of the women and 13% of the men had used analgesics. The most significant predictor of analgesic use was headache; a lesser association was found with infections. Drug use in women was associated with symptoms of depression. Drug use in men was associated with sleeplessness. Higher drug use was associated with smoking and high coffee consumption, but not with frequent alcohol intake [29].

Patients attending an outpatient neurology clinic in Austria reported taking, on average, 6.3 different headache pain drugs [30]. Of these patients, 26.5% reported using both prescription and over-the-counter medications; 31.3% used over-the-counter medications only, and 27.7% used prescription drugs only. Acetaminophen (paracetamol; average dose 500 mg) was the most frequently used analgesic. Most patients attending a London migraine clinic used multiple medications [31]. Again acetaminophen was the most commonly used analgesic (34.9%), followed by aspirin (22.9%).

How common is MOH? This is uncertain, since some cases are drug-induced and some are just associated with drug overuse. In European headache centers, 5–10% of patients have MOH. One series of 3000 consecutive headache patients reported that 4.3% had MOH [32]. In US specialty headache clinics, as many as 80% of patients who presented with daily or near-daily headache used analgesics on a daily or near-daily basis [21]. In other headache clinics a smaller percentage, although still a majority, are reported to have the problem [33]. In contrast, medication overuse is less common in India [34].

Diener and Dahlöf [24] summarized 29 studies that included 2612 patients with MOH. Sixty-five percent of patients had migraine as their primary headache, 27% tension-type headache (TTH), and 8% mixed or other headaches (i.e., cluster headache). Women had more MOH than men (3.5:1; 1533 women, 442 men). The mean duration of primary headache was 20.4 years. The mean admitted time of frequent drug intake was 10.3 years in one study, and the mean duration of daily headache was 5.9 years. Patients averaged 2.5 to 5.8 different pharmacologic components simultaneously (range 1 to 14) [24]. Patients who overused triptans took fewer doses per day [35]. It is our belief that MOH can only occur with a substrate of migraine. TTH in the past would probably be reclassified as migraine or probable migraine.

In population-based epidemiologic studies, approximately 1–2% of the general population have MOH [36–39]. Moreover, MOH is a growing problem in Asian countries, such as China and Taiwan [38], with the same prevalence as that observed in Europe. MOH occurs in early adolescence and childhood [40], as early as age 6 years [41]. One Taiwanese study revealed a prevalence of chronic daily headache in a population of adolescents (12 to 14 years of age) of 1.5%. Only 20% of them overused acute headache medication, confirming previous findings that medication overuse is less important in children and adolescents [42].

A random telephone survey of 24,159 households in Canada produced a sample of 1573 households with one or more eligible headache sufferers. Ninety percent of the ICHD-diagnosed migraineurs reported using over-the-counter drugs and 44% reported using prescription drugs. In this sample, 1.5% of migraineurs had MOH resulting from ergotamine tartrate or analgesic overuse [43].

In the past, MOH was usually due to the overuse of analgesics, barbiturates, opioids or ergots. Now triptans have became widely used and overused. A Danish prescription register study found that the prevalence of sumatriptan use in 1995 was 0.78%. Of these, up to 5% overused sumatriptan on a daily basis [44]. Evers and colleagues found that 4.7% of 320 sumatriptan users overused the drug by taking it at least every other day [45].

Pathophysiology

Medication overuse headache is primarily a complication of migraine. Non-migraineurs who overuse acute medication do not develop MOH [46]. MOH only occurs in cluster headache patients who have coexistent migraine. Migraineurs who take analgesics for treatment of non-headache pain conditions are significantly more likely to develop MOH than are non-migraineurs [47].

The mammalian nervous system contains networks that modulate nociceptive transmission. A descending inhibitory neuronal network extends from the frontal cortex and hypothalamus through the periaqueductal gray (PAG) to the rostral ventromedial medulla (RVM) and the medullary and spinal dorsal horn. In the RVM and PAG, three classes of neurons ('off-cells', 'on-cells' and neutral cells) exist [48]. Off-cells pause immediately before the nociceptive reflex, whereas on-cells are activated. Neutral cells show no consistent changes in activation [49]. Opioids activate off-cells and inhibit on-cells; and nociceptive reflexes are inhibited. Opioid withdrawal results in increased on-cell activity, decreased off-cell activity, and enhanced nociception [48,50–51]. Thus, off-cell activity suppresses nociception, whereas on-cell activity enhances the response to noxious stimuli.

The RVM modulates trigeminal nucleus caudalis (TNC) activity. Descending facilitatory influences could contribute to chronic pain states and the development and maintenance of hyperalgesia [52]. Acute medication (analgesics, opioids, barbiturates, ergotamine-containing compounds or triptans) overuse [53] could result in resetting the pain control mechanisms in susceptible individuals, perhaps by enhancing on-cell activity, enhancing central sensitization through N-methyl-D-aspartate (NMDA) receptors, or blocking adaptive antinociceptive changes.

Opioids can induce pain and decrease tolerance to nociception. This is similar to the pathologic pain that follows peripheral nerve injury. Both activate the RVM descending pain facilitation pathways. Opioid analgesic tolerance is, in part, due to activation of the NMDA receptor (NMDAR). Excess activation of NMDARs can lead to neurotoxicity. Opioid-induced neurotoxicity depletes inhibitory GABA (gamma-aminobutyric acid) interneurons, a mechanism that may have clinical implications in opioid therapy and substance abuse and may account for refractoriness in MOH.

Central sensitization, defined by the presence of cutaneous allodynia, exists in chronic daily headache (CDH), including MOH. Shukla et al. [54] found that dynamic mechanical (brush) allodynia (BA) is common in hospitalized CDH patients. Of a total of 78 patients, most of whom had transformed migraine (TM), 32 (41%) experienced BA. Creach et al. [55] compared heat-pain thresholds in patients with TM with and without medication overuse and patients with episodic migraine. Extracranial, but not face, allodynia was more common in both TM groups (39.5% vs 12.1%). Using a questionnaire, Sobrino [56] found that 56.3% of TM patients had cutaneous allodynia in their pain-referred areas. Ayzenberg et al. simultaneously recorded blink reflex and nociceptive cortical potentials following nociceptive trigeminal stimulation. They demonstrated a temporary facilitation of the trigeminal nociceptive system at a supraspinal level, which normalized after withdrawal [57].

Chronic substance exposure can induce changes in receptor expression and sensitization. Chronic application of non-opioid analgesics in rats significantly decreased the number of 5-HT2A binding sites and increased the number of 5-HT (5-hydroxytryptamine; serotonin) transporter binding sites in the CNS [58]. Reuter et al. studied 5-HT receptor expression and function in rats following chronic application of sumatriptan and zolmitriptan. Their regular (daily) exposure to 5-HT$_{1B/D}$ produced significant downregulation in 5-HT$_{1B/D}$ receptors in various cortical regions, the extrapyramidal system and the brainstem, and influenced the serotonin synthesis rate [59,60]. Downregulation of 5-HT receptors may occur as early as 24 to 96 hours following chronic exposure [61]. This may lead to a downregulation of 5-HT receptors and change central inhibitory pathways.

Imaging studies provide insights into the pathophysiology of MOH. One study investigated glucose metabolism in 16 MOH patients before and after withdrawal compared with 68 healthy controls. They found reversible hypometabolic changes in brain regions belonging to the general pain network. The orbitofrontal cortex continued to show persistent hypometabolism before and after drug withdrawal, more so when patients were overusing combination analgesics [62].

Diagnosis

Medication overuse headache should be ruled out in all patients with CDH or very frequent headaches; but it is frequently overlooked. Ask patients what they are taking for their headache, not what medications they are taking, because they often forget to mention over-the-counter analgesics. Several clinical characteristics may help identify MOH in patients with very frequent or daily headache disorders (Table 7.2)[4].

In a German prospective study of 98 patients [63,64], triptan overuse outnumbered ergot overuse. Migraine patients with triptan-induced

Table 7.2 Characteristics of medication overuse headache.

General headache symptoms and observations	The headaches are refractory, daily, or nearly daily
	The pain often varies in severity, type and location
	Withdrawal symptoms occur when the patient's acute medication is abruptly stopped
	Spontaneous headache improvement often occurs when the overused medications are discontinued
	Concomitant prophylactic medications may be ineffective while the patients are overusing acute medication
Associated symptoms	Asthenia, nausea, gastrointestinal symptoms
	Comorbid mood disorder
	Memory problems and difficulty in concentration
Special symptoms under ergot overuse	Cold extremities, tachycardia, paresthesias, 'irritable bowl syndrome'
	Diminished pulse, hypertension, light-headedness, muscle pain of the extremities, weakness of the legs

headache not only developed a migraine-like daily headache, but also a significant increase in migraine attack frequency. The delay between the medication overuse and the development of daily headache was shortest for triptans (1.7 years), longer for ergots (2.7 years), and longest for analgesics (4.8 years). The intake frequency (single dosages per month) was lowest for triptans (18 single dosages per month), higher for ergots (37 single dosages per month), and highest for analgesics (114 single dosages per month). Triptans not only cause a different spectrum of clinical features, but are able to cause MOH faster and with lower dosages than other substance groups [25].

Management

Patients with MOH, especially when complicated by comorbid psychiatric disease, low frustration tolerance, and physical and emotional dependency, can be difficult to treat [65,66]. We start patients on preventive medication with the understanding that the drugs may not become fully effective until medication overuse has been eliminated [31]. Some patients remain refractory [67] and need to be detoxified and/or have their headache cycle terminated.

Patients need education and continuous support. Disturbances in mood and function are common and require management with behavioral methods of pain management and supportive psychotherapy. It is often necessary to treat coexistent psychiatric illness before MOH comes under control. Chronobiologic interventions, such as encouraging regular habits of sleep, exercise and meals, can be useful [31].

The following principles guide the use of preventive treatment:

1 Choose a preventive agent based on its adverse event (AE) profiles, comorbid and coexistent conditions, and specific indications.
2 Start at a low dose.
3 Gradually increase the dose until you achieve efficacy, the patient develops side effects, or the ceiling dose for the drug in question is reached.
4 Treatment effects develop over weeks and treatment may not become fully effective until rebound is eliminated.
5 If one agent fails and if all other factors are equal, choose an agent from another therapeutic class.
6 Prefer monotherapy, but be willing to use combination therapy.
7 Communicate realistic expectations [68].

Most preventive agents used for primary CDH/MOH have not been examined in well-designed double-blind studies. Table 7.3 summarizes an assessment of the efficacy, safety and evidence for a number of agents [31]. Topiramate's efficacy in treating chronic migraine (CM) was recently demonstrated in two prospective, double-blind, randomized, placebo-controlled studies done in the USA [69] and Europe [70]. A key difference between the US and European trials was that patients were allowed to take acute rescue medication as usual during the European trial. The benefits of topiramate were seen in the subgroup of patients overusing acute

Table 7.3 Summary of prophylactic drugs for use in chronic daily headache/medication overuse headache.

Drug	Clinical efficacy	Adverse events	Clinical evidence
Antidepressants			
Amitriptyline	+++	++	+++
Doxepin	+++	++	++
Fluoxetine	++	+	+++
Anticonvulsants			
Divalproex	+++	++	++
Gabapentin	++	++	+++
Topiramate	++++	++	+++
Beta-blockers			
Propranolol, nadolol, etc.	++	+	+

medications (MOH) in the absence of detoxification. This provided evidence that topiramate reduces headache frequency even in migraine patients with chronic migraine who are overusing medication [70]. This result was partially replicated in protocol violators in a second trial [69]. This, in part, negates the belief that medical and behavioral headache treatment may fail as long as the patient continues to overuse acute medication.

MOH can revert to episodic headache when preventive medication is initiated and acute medications limited. In other cases, there may be only moderate or no improvement. Zeeberg et al. studied 337 patients with MOH. A 46% decrease in headache frequency from the first visit to dismissal occurred ($p < 0.0001$). Patients with no improvement 2 months after complete drug withdrawal ($n = 88$) subsequently responded to pharmacologic and/or non-pharmacologic prophylaxis, with a 26% decrease in headache frequency as measured from the end of withdrawal to dismissal. At dismissal, 47% of patients were on prophylaxis. In this population, about half of MOH patients benefit from drug withdrawal alone [71].

Patients can have severe migraine exacerbation during detoxification. Thus patients, even if they are on preventive medication, often need additional treatment (which we call *headache terminators*) to break the cycle of daily headache and/or help with the exacerbation that occurs when overused medications are discontinued. Terminators can be given orally, by suppository or by injection, and some can be given intravenously repetitively. The route of administration depends on both the setting and the intensity of treatment.

Typical withdrawal symptoms last for 2 to 10 days (average 3.5 days) and include severely exacerbated headaches accompanied by nausea, vomiting, agitation, restlessness, sleep disorder and (rarely) seizures. Barbiturates, opioids and benzodiazepine, unless replaced with long-acting derivatives, must be tapered to avoid serious withdrawal symptoms. The withdrawal phase is much shorter when patients are abusing only triptans. The vulnerable period may last 3 to 8 weeks; once it is over, considerable

Table 7.4 Outpatient or inpatient withdrawal therapy.

Outpatient	Patient highly motivated and self-disciplined
	Patient overuses triptans or simple analgesics. No combinations or use of barbiturates, opioids or tranquilizers
	Severe signs or side effects of medication overuse are absent (ergotism, peptic ulcers, sleep disturbances)
	No coexistent psychiatric disease of sufficient severity such that a failure to admit could pose a health risk to the patient or impair the implementation of outpatient treatment
Hospitalization	Failed outpatient withdrawal
	Overuse of barbiturates, tranquilizers, or opioids
	Coexistent or risk of disease necessitating monitoring for treatment of headache significant enough to warrant admission
	Complications of overuse such as ergotism, peptic ulcers, diarrhea, anemia
	Coexistent psychiatric disorder of sufficient severity

headache improvement frequently occurs [4,18,72,73]. Patients with MOH may not become fully responsive to acute and preventive treatment for 2 to 10 weeks after medication overuse is eliminated, and some may never fully respond.

Drug withdrawal is performed in different ways. Treatment in an ambulatory infusion unit and home treatment are two outpatient options. They are suited for patients who take simple analgesics not containing barbiturates or opioids. If outpatient treatment proves difficult or is dangerous, hospitalization may be required (Table 7.4) [74,75]. Diener et al. [76] were able to detoxify only 1.5% of 200 patients on an outpatient basis. Hering and Steiner [77], in contrast, successfully used outpatient detoxification for 37 of 46 patients who were taking simple analgesics or ergotamine. They abruptly withdrew the offending drugs, utilizing adequate explanation of the disorder, regular follow-up, and amitriptyline (10 mg at night) and naproxen (500 mg) for relief of headache symptoms. The German Migraine Society consensus paper [78] recommends outpatient withdrawal for patients who do not take barbiturates or tranquilizers with their analgesics and are highly motivated. Patients who fail outpatient treatment or have a high depression score require inpatient treatment.

We believe hospitalization is necessary when the following conditions are present:

- severe dehydration, for which inpatient parenteral therapy may be necessary;
- prolonged, unrelenting headache with associated symptoms, such as nausea and vomiting, which, if allowed to continue, would pose a further threat to the patient's welfare;
- dependence on mixed analgesics, ergots, opioids, barbiturates or tranquilizers;
- pain that is accompanied by serious adverse reactions or complications from therapy wherein continued use of such therapy aggravates or induces further illness;

- pain that occurs in the presence of significant medical disease but appropriate treatment of headache symptom aggravates or induces further illness;
- failed outpatient detoxification, for which inpatient pain and psychiatric management may be necessary;
- treatment requiring co-pharmacy with drugs that may cause a drug interaction, thus necessitating careful observation (monoamine oxidase inhibitors and beta-blockers) (Table 7.4).

Two general detoxification strategies are in use. One approach is to taper the overused medication. The alternative strategy is to abruptly discontinue the overused drug, substitute a transitional medication to replace the overused drug, and subsequently taper the transitional drug. If high doses of a butalbital-containing analgesic combination are abruptly discontinued, phenobarbital should be used to control barbiturate withdrawal symptoms. Similarly, benzodiazepines must be gradually tapered or replaced with long-acting ones. Ergotamine can be replaced with dihydroergotamine (DHE) and short-acting non-steroidal anti-inflammatory drugs (NSAIDs) with long-acting ones. Terminators are used to stop the headache cycle (see below). Patients who do not need hospital-level care but cannot be safely or adequately treated at home can be considered for ambulatory infusion treatment. It is best done in a supervised medical setting where the patient can be monitored frequently (every 15 minutes). Under these circumstances, repetitive intravenous treatment can be given twice a day for several days in a row.

The goals of inpatient headache treatment include: (i) detoxification; (ii) rehydration; (iii) pain control with headache termination; (iv) establishment of effective preventive treatment; (v) patient education; and (vi) establishment of outpatient methods of pain control [67]. In the hospital, simple analgesics can be stopped abruptly. Barbiturates, opioids and benzodiazepine, unless replaced with long-acting derivatives, must be tapered to avoid a serious withdrawal syndrome. Fluids should given, especially if severe nausea or vomiting is present. Vomiting can be treated with antiemetics or neuroleptics. Butalbital withdrawal can be treated with phenobarbital [60–100 mg i.v. (intravenously) or i.m. (intramuscularly)] as needed. Opioid withdrawal can be treated with methadone replacement. Milder symptoms can be treated with clonidine (0.1–0.2 mg t.i.d. titrated up or down based on withdrawal symptoms). Some patients may require anxiolytic medication. Behavioral techniques, such as relaxation-therapy and stress management, are useful.

Patients often need *headache terminators* to break the cycle of daily headache and/or help with the exacerbation that occurs when overused medications are discontinued. Terminators are given orally, by suppository or by injection, and some – DHE, neuroleptics (prochlorperazine, chlorpromazine and droperidol), corticosteroids, valproate sodium, magnesium and ketorolac – can be given repetitively intravenously. Outpatient home terminators include long-acting NSAIDs, Cox-2 inhibitors, short courses of corticosteroids, and typical (e.g., prochlorperazine suppositories) and atypical (e.g. olanzapine) neuroleptics. We teach patients to self-inject DHE (subcutaneous or intramuscular DHE; 0.25–1 mg), ketorolac and droperidol. Valproate has been shown to have beneficial effects in the preventive treatment of CDH complicated by excessive analgesic intake [79]. A recent, large, open trial showed that cortisone effectively reduces withdrawal symptoms, including rebound headache [80]. A double-blind study showed a single subcutaneous dose of sumatriptan to be better than placebo in the treatment of ergotamine withdrawal headache, but the headache reappeared within 12 hours [81]. An open randomized study indicated that naproxen was better than symptomatic treatment with antiemetics and analgesics [82].

Some experts delay preventive treatment until withdrawal is completed. If a patient then experiences more than three migraine attacks a month, they introduce medical and behavioral prophylaxis. Patients may respond to preventive treatment after drug withdrawal despite the fact that these drugs had been unsuccessful before. Is this the effect of detoxification or the result of terminating the headache cycle?

Prevention

It is most important that patients receive proper instruction and appropriate surveillance. At risk are migraineurs with high-frequency headaches. Acute medication should be limited and preventive treatment started.

Ergotamine and triptan use must be restricted (no more than twice per week) [25]. Drugs that contain barbiturates, caffeine, codeine or tranquilizers, as well as mixed analgesics, should be limited. Patients who take over-the-counter medication should be advised to limit caffeine combinations. A headache diary can help detect increased attack frequency or medication usage as early as possible. Early migraine prevention, either by medical or behavioral treatment, can help avoid MOH.

Prognosis

The mean success rate of withdrawal therapy over 1–6 months is 72.4% (17 studies, $n = 1101$ patients). Success is defined as at least an improvement of more than 50% in headache days. Three older studies (pre-triptan era) had longer observation periods (between 9 and 35 months) [18,83,84]. The success rates in these studies were 60%, 70% and 73%, respectively. A 5-year follow-up study found a relapse rate of 40% [84]. Recent studies included patients with triptan-induced MOH [85–87]. The relapse rate for the first year after successful withdrawal therapy was 38%, and about 42% after 4 years in two studies [85,87]. Patients are at greatest risk of relapse within the first

12 months, but have a lower risk of relapsing 12 months after withdrawal. Patients who initially overused analgesics (mostly combination analgesics) had higher relapse rates than patients who overused ergots or triptans (58% vs 22% vs 19%, respectively, for the first 12 months). Other predictors, such as duration of drug overuse, duration of disorder, and presence of prophylactic treatment, did not influence the relapse rate, either within the first 12 months or within 48 months [87].

Over 600 consecutive migraine patients without MOH or CDH were prospectively followed for 12 months [88]. Fourteen percent of this cohort developed CDH within one year, and two-thirds, or almost 10%, of these patients fulfilled the criteria of MOH. Two main predictors could be identified: (i) a high initial frequency of headache events; and (ii) medication overuse. This confirms findings from population-based studies suggesting that analgesic overuse predicted the persistence of CDH [38,89]. In one of the few prospective population-based studies, Zwart et al. [90] showed that analgesic overuse strongly predicted chronic pain associated with analgesic overuse 11 years later, particularly among those with chronic migraine. Analgesic overuse is significantly more strongly associated with chronic headache than with other chronic pain conditions, such as chronic neck pain or chronic low back pain [91].

References

1 Katsarava Z, Limmroth V, Fritsche G, Diener HC. Drug-induced headache following the use of zolmitriptan or naratriptan. Cephalalgia 1999;19:414 [abstract].

2 Saper JR, Jones JM. Ergotamine tartrate dependency: features and possible mechanisms. Clin Neuropharmacol 1986;9:244–56.

3 Silberstein SD, Lipton RB, Solomon S, Mathew NT. Classification of daily and near daily headaches: proposed revisions to the IHS classification. Headache 1994;34:1–7.

4 Mathew NT, Kurman R, Perez F. Drug induced refractory headache – clinical features and management. Headache 1990;30:634–8.

5 Mathew NT. Drug induced headache. Neurol Clin 1990; 8:903–12.

6 Diamond S, Dalessio DJ. Drug abuse in headache. In: Diamond S, Dalessio DJ (eds) The Practicing Physician's Approach to Headache, 3rd edn. Baltimore: Lippincott, Williams & Wilkins, 1982;114–21.

7 Wilkinson M. Introduction. In: Diener HC, Wilkinson M (eds) Drug-Induced Headache. Berlin: Springer-Verlag, 1988;1–2.

8 Saper JR. Ergotamine dependence. Headache 1987;27:435–8.

9 Saper JR. Chronic headache syndromes. Neurol Clin 1989; 7:387–412.

10 Mihatsch MJ. Das Analgetikasyndrom. Stuttgart, New York: Thieme, 1986.

11 Peters G, Horton BT. Headache: with special reference to the excessive use of ergotamine preparations and withdrawal effects. Proc Mayo Clin 1951;26:153–61.

12 Horton BT, Peters GA. Clinical manifestations of excessive use of ergotamine preparations and management of withdrawal effect: report of 52 cases. Headache 1963;3:214–26.

13 Diener HC, Wilkinson M. Drug-Induced Headache. Berlin, Heidelberg, New York: Springer, 2004.

14 Diener HC, Limmroth V. Medication-overuse headache: a worldwide problem. Lancet Neurol 2004;3:475–83.

15 Kaube H, May A, Diener HC, Pfaffenrath V. Sumatriptan misuse in daily chronic headache. Br Med J 1994;308:1573.

16 Limmroth V, Kazarawa S, Fritsche G, Diener HC. Headache after frequent use of new 5-HT agonists zolmitriptan and naratriptan. Lancet 1999;353:378.

17 Andersson PG. Ergotism: the clinical picture. In: Diener HC, Wilkinson MS (eds) Drug-Induced Headache. Berlin: Springer, 1988: 16–19.

18 Baumgartner C, Wessly P, Bingol C, et al. Long-term prognosis of analgesic withdrawal in patients with drug-induced headaches. Headache 1989;29:510–14.

19 Rapoport AM, Weeks RE, Sheftell FD, Baskin SM, Verdi J. The "analgesic washout period": a critical variable evaluation in the evaluation of headache treatment efficacy. Neurology 1986;36:100–1.

20 Dichgans J, Diener HD, Gerber WD, et al. Analgetika-induzierter dauerkopfschmerz. Dtsch Med Wschr 1984;109:369.

21 Rapoport AM. Analgesic rebound headache. Headache 1988;28:662–5.

22 Headache Classification Committee. The International Classification of Headache Disorders, 2nd Edition. Cephalalgia 2004;24:1–160.

23 Saper JR. Headache Disorders: Current Concepts in Treatment Strategies. Littleton: Wright-PSG, 1983.

24 Diener HC, Dahlöf CG. Headache associated with chronic use of substances. In: Olesen J, Tfelt-Hansen P, Welch KMA (eds) The Headaches, 2nd edn. Philadelphia: Lippincott, Williams & Wilkins, 1999;871–8.

25 Limmroth V, Katsarava Z, Fritsche G, Przywara S, Diener HC. Features of medication overuse headache following overuse of different acute headache drugs. Neurology 2002;59:1011–14.

26 Gutzwiller F, Zemp E. Der analgetikakonsum in der bevölkerung und socioökonomische aspekte des analgetikaabusus. In: Mihatsch MJ (ed.) Das Analgetikasyndrom. Stuttgart: Thieme, 1986;197–205.

27 Kieholz P, Ladewig D. Probleme des medikamentenmissbrauches. Schweis Arztezeitung 1981;62:2866–9.

28 Schwarz A, Farber U, Glaeske G. Daten zu analgetikakonsum and analgetikanephropathie in der bundesrepublik. Offentiches gesundheitswesen 1985;47:298–300.

29 Eggen AE. The Tromsø study: frequency and predicting factors of analgesic drug use in a free-living population (12–56 years). J Clin Epidemiol 1993;46:1297–304.

30 Schnider P, Aull S, Feucht M. Use and abuse of analgesics in tension-type headache. Cephalalgia 1994;14:162–7.

31 Silberstein SD, Saper JR. Migraine: diagnosis and treatment. In: Dalessio DJ, Silberstein SD (eds) Wolff's Headache and other Head Pain, 6th edn. New York: Oxford University Press, 1993; 96–170.

32 Micieli G, Manzoni GC, Granella F, Martignoni E, Malferrari G, Nappi G. Clinical and epidemiological observations on drug abuse in headache patients. In: Diener HC, Wilkinson M (eds) Drug-Induced Headache. Berlin: Springer-Verlag, 1988; 20–8.

33 Solomon S, Lipton RB, Newman LC. Clinical features of chronic daily headache. Headache 1992;32:325–9.

34 Ravishankar K. Headache pattern in India: A headache clinic analysis of 1000 patients. Cephalalgia 1997;17:143–4.

35 IHS. Draft International Headache Society Classification. 2002. Available at: www.I-H-S.org.

36 Tekle Haimanot R, Seraw B, Forsgren L, Ekbom K, Ekstedt J. Migraine, chronic tension-type headache, and cluster headache in an Ethiopian rural community. Cephalalgia 1995;15:482–8.

37 Castillo J, Munoz P, Guitera V, Pascual J. Epidemiology of chronic daily headache in the general population. Headache 1999;39:190–6.

38 Wang SJ, Fuh JL, Lu SR, et al. Chronic daily headache in Chinese elderly: prevalence, risk factors and biannual follow-up. Neurology 2000;54:314–19.

39 Scher AI, Stewart WF, Liberman J, Lipton RB. Prevalence of frequent headache in a population sample. Headache 1998;38:497–506.

40 Hershey AD. Chronic daily headaches in children. Expert Opin Pharmacother 2003;4:485–91.

41 Hering-Hanit R, Gadoth N, Cohen A, Horev Z. Successful withdrawal from analgesic abuse in a group of youngsters with chronic daily headache. J Child Neurol 2001;16:448–9.

42 Wang SJ, Fuh JL, Lu SR, Juang KD. Chronic daily headache in adolescents: prevalence, impact, and medication overuse. Neurology 2006;66:193–7.

43 Robinson RG. Pain relief for headaches. Can Fam Physician 1993;39: 867–72.

44 Gaist D, Hallas J, Sindrup SH, Gram LF. Is overuse of sumatriptan a problem? A population-based study. Eur J Clin Pharmacol 1996;50:161–5.

45 Evers S, Suhr B, Bauer B, Grotemeyer KH, Husstedt IW. A retrospective long-term analysis of the epidemiology and features of drug-induced headache. J Neurol 1999;246:802–9.

46 Lance F, Parkes C, Wilkinson M. Does analgesic abuse cause headache de novo? Headache 1988;1:61–2.

47 Bahra A, Walsh M, Menon S, Goadsby PJ. Does chronic daily headache arise de novo in association with regular analgesic use? Cephalalgia 2000;20:294 [abstract].

48 Fields HL, Heinricher MM, Mason P. Neurotransmitters as nociceptive modulatory circuits. Ann Rev Neurosci 1991;219–45.

49 Messlinger K, Burstein R. Anatomy of central nervous system pathways related to head pain. In: Olesen J, Tfelt-Hansen P, Welch KMA (eds) The Headaches, 2nd edn. Philadelphia: Lippincott, Williams & Wilkins, 1999;77.

50 Kim DH, Fields HL, Barbaro NM. Morphine analgesia and acute physical dependence: rapid onset of two opposing, dose-related processes. Brain Res 1990;516:37–40.

51 Bederson JB, Fields HL, Barbaro NM. Hyperalgesia during naloxone-precipitated withdrawal from morphine is associated with increased on-cell activity in the rostral ventromedial medulla. Somatosens Mot Res 1990;7: 185–203.

52 Urban MO, Gebhart GF. Supraspinal contributions to hyperalgesia. Proc Natl Acad Sci USA 1999;96:7687–92.

53 Post RM, Silberstein SD. Shared mechanisms in affective illness, epilepsy, and migraine. Neurology 1994;44:S37–S47.

54 Shukla P, Richardson E, Young WB. Brush allodynia in an inpatient headache unit. Headache 2003;43:542 [abstract].

55 Creach C, Radat F, Laffitau M, Irachabal S, Henry P. Cutaneous allodynia in transformed migraine with medication overuse. Cephalalgia 2003;23:656 [abstract].

56 Sobrino FE. Cutaneous allodynia in chronic migraine. Cephalalgia 2003;23:750 [abstract].

57 Ayzenberg I, Obermann M, Nyhuis P, et al. Central sensitization of the trigeminal and somatic nociceptive systems in medication overuse headache mainly involves cerebral supraspinal structures. Cephalalgia 2006;26:1106–14.

58 Srikiatkhachorn A, Tarasub N, Govitrapong P. Effect of chronic analgesic exposure on the central serotonin system: a possible mechanism of analgesic abuse headache. Headache 2000;40:343–50.

59 Dobson CF, Tohyama Y, Diksic M, Hamel E. Effects of acute or chronic administration of anti-migraine drugs sumatriptan and zolmitriptan on serotonin synthesis in the rat brain. Cephalalgia 2004;24:2–11.

60 Reuter U, Salomone S, Ickenstein GW, Waeber C. Effects of chronic sumatriptan and zolmitriptan treatment on 5-HT receptor expression and function in rats. Cephalalgia 2004;24:398–407.

61 Saucier C, Morris SJ, Albert PR. Endogenous serotonin-2A and -2C receptors in Balb/c-3T3 cells revealed in serotonin-free medium: desensitization and down-regulation by serotonin. Biochem Pharmacol 1998;56:1347–57.

62 Fumal A, Laureys S, Di CL, et al. Orbitofrontal cortex involvement in chronic analgesic-overuse headache evolving from episodic migraine. Brain 2006;129:543–50.

63 Katsarava Z, Fritsche G, Diener HC, Limmroth V. Drug-induced headache (DIH): following the use of different triptans. Cephalalgia 2000;20:293 [abstract].

64 Diener HC, Katsarava Z. Analgesic/abortive overuse and misuse in chronic daily headache. Curr Pain Headache Rep 2001;5:545–50.

65 Mathew NT, Reuveni U, Perez F. Transformed or evolutive migraine. Headache 1987;27:102–6.

66 Saper JR. Ergotamine dependency – a review. Headache 1987;27:435–8.

67 Saper JR, Lake AE, III, Madden SF, Kreeger C. Comprehensive/tertiary care for headache: a 6-month outcome study. Headache 1999;39:249–63.

68 Silberstein SD, Lipton RB. Overview of diagnosis and treatment of migraine. Neurology 1994;44:6–16.

69 Silberstein SD, Lipton RB, Dodick DW, et al. Efficacy and safety of topiramate for the treatment of chronic migraine: a randomized, double-blind, placebo-controlled trial. Headache 2007;47:170–80.

70 Diener HC, Bussone G, Van Oene JC, Lahaye M, Schwalen S, Goadsby PJ. Topiramate reduces headache days in chronic migraine: a randomized, double-blind, placebo-controlled study. Cephalalgia 2007;27:814–23.

71 Zeeberg P, Olesen J, Jensen R. Discontinuation of medication overuse in headache patients: recovery of therapeutic responsiveness. Cephalalgia 2006;26:1192–8.

72 Silberstein SD, Schulman EA, Hopkins MM. Repetitive intravenous DHE in the treatment of refractory headache. Headache 1990;30:334–9.

73 Raskin NH. Repetitive intravenous dihydroergotamine as therapy for intractable migraine. Neurology 1986;36:995–7.

74 Saper JR, Silberstein SD, Gordon CD, Hamel RL, Swidan S. Handbook of Headache Management: A Practical Guide to Diagnosis and Treatment of Head, Neck, and Facial Pain, 2nd edn. Baltimore: Lippincott, Williams & Wilkins, 1999.

75 Lake AE, Saper JR, Hamel RL. Inpatient treatment of intractable headache: outcome for 267 consecutive program completers. Headache 2006;46:893 [abstract].

76 Diener HC, Gerber WD, Geiselhart S. Short and long-term effects of withdrawal therapy in drug-induced headache. In: Diener HC, Wilkinson M (eds) Drug-Induced Headache. Berlin: Springer-Verlag, 1988; 133–42.

77 Hering R, Steiner TJ. Abrupt outpatient withdrawal from medication in analgesic-abusing migraineurs. Lancet 1991;337:1442–3.

78 Haag G, Baar H, Grotemeyer KH, Pfaffenrath V, Ribbat MJ, Diener HC. [Prophylaxis and treatment of drug-induced persistent headache. Therapy recommendation of the German Society for Migraine and Headache]. Schmerz 1999;13:52–7.

79 Mathew NT, Ali S. Valproate in the treatment of persistent chronic daily headache. An open label study. Headache 1991;31:71–4.

80 Krymchantowski AV, Barbosa JS. Prednisone as initial treatment of analgesic-induced daily headache. Cephalalgia 2000;20:107–13.

81 Diener HC, Haab J, Peters C, Ried S, Dichgans J, Pilgrim A. Subcutaneous sumatriptan in the treatment of headache during withdrawal from drug-induced headache. Headache 1991;31:205–9.

82 Mathew NT. Amelioration of ergotamine withdrawal symptoms with naproxen. Headache 1987;27:130–3.

83 Diener HC, Dichgans J, Scholz E, Geiselhart S, Gerber WD, Bille A. Analgesic-induced chronic headache: long-term results of withdrawal therapy. J Neurol 1989;236:9–14.

84 Schnider P, Aull S, Baumgartner C, et al. Long-term outcome of patients with headache and drug abuse after inpatient withdrawal: five-year followup. Cephalalgia 1996;16:481–5.

85 Katsarava Z, Muebig M, Fritsche G, Diener HC, Limmroth V. Clinical features of withdrawal headache following overuse of triptans in comparison to other antiheadache drugs. Neurology 2001;57:1694–8.

86 Fritsche G, Eberl A, Katsarava Z, Limmroth V, Diener HC. Drug-induced headache: long-term follow-up of withdrawal therapy and persistence of drug misuse. Eur Neurol 2001;45:229–35.

87 Katsarava Z, Limmroth V, Finke M, Diener HC, Fritsche G. Rates and predictors for relapse in medication overuse headache: a 1-year prospective study. Neurology 2003;60:1682–3.

88 Katsarava Z, Schneeweiss S, Kurth T, et al. Incidence and predictors for chronicity of headache in patients with episodic migraine. Neurology 2004;62:788–90.

89 Lu SR, Fuh JL, Chen WT, Juan KD, Wang SJ. Chronic daily headache in Taipei, Taiwan: prevalence, follow-up and outcome predictors. Cephalalgia 2001;21:980–6.

90 Zwart JA, Dyb G, Hagen K, Svebak S, Holmen J. Analgesic use: a predictor of chronic pain and medication overuse headache: the Head-HUNT Study. Neurology 2003;61:160–4.

91 Zwart JA, Dyb G, Hagen K, Svebak S, Stovner LJ, Holmen J. Analgesic overuse among subjects with headache, neck, and low-back pain. Neurology 2004;62:1540–4.
92 Headache Classification Committee of the International Headache Society. Classification and diagnostic criteria for headache disorders, cranial neuralgia, and facial pain. Cephalalgia 1988;8:1–96.

8 Migraine and Other Comorbidities: Obesity, Temporomandibular Disorders and Contact Points

Marcelo E. Bigal

Merck Research Laboratories, Whitehouse Station, NJ, USA; and Department of Neurology, Albert Einstein College of Medicine, NY, USA

Introduction

The term 'comorbidity', coined by Feinstein, is now widely used to refer to the greater than coincidental association of two conditions in the same individual [1,2]. Migraine has been noted to be comorbid with a number of other illnesses in specialty care and in population samples [3,4]. Understanding the comorbidity of migraine is potentially important from a number of different perspectives. Migraine could be comorbid with other conditions due to diagnostic uncertainty and overlapping symptom profiles. For example, both migraine and epilepsy can cause transient alterations of consciousness as well as headache [5]. The migraine aura shares some of the features of stroke or transient ischemic attack. Other conditions may arise as sequelae of repeated attacks. For example, medication side effects and subclinical infarcts (see below) may increase with lifetime attack frequency [6]. Finally, the study of comorbidity may provide epidemiologic or biological clues to the fundamental mechanisms of migraine.

Historically, a number of conditions have been noted to be comorbid with migraine, notably psychiatric disorders (anxiety, depression, panic disorder), epilepsy, asthma and some congenital heart defects. These are topics of specific chapters in this book. In this chapter we focus on some less frequently discussed comorbidities. We specifically focus on the relationship between migraine and obesity, temporomandibular disorders and intranasal contact points. For each of these comorbidities, we first discuss the evidence linking each of them with migraine, and then briefly discuss clinical interventions for each comorbid disorder.

Comorbidity in Migraine, First Edition. Edited by J. Schoenen, D. W. Dodick and P. S. Sándor.
© 2011 Blackwell Publishing Ltd. Published 2011 by Blackwell Publishing Ltd.

Obesity

Much interest has been paid to the relationship between obesity and primary headaches. This is partially driven by the fact that most preventive medications typically used to treat migraine have the potential for weight gain, in addition to the fact that both migraine and obesity seem to be a risk factor for cardiovascular disorders [7,8].

While most studies have failed to demonstrate a comorbid relationship between episodic migraine and obesity [9–11], it is well established that obesity is a risk factor for increased headache attacks among migraineurs (and therefore a risk factor for chronic migraine). This relationship has now been explored in four large population studies. In the first study, Scher and colleagues [12] followed individuals with episodic headaches over the course of one year and found that 3% progressed to chronic daily headaches (CDH). Among the risk factors for progression, obesity figured prominently; the relative odds of CDH were five times higher in individuals with a body mass index (BMI) ≥30, than in those with normal bodyweight. Overweight individuals (BMI ranging from 25 to 29) had a three-fold increased risk of developing CDH. In the cross-sectional component of the study it was found that obesity was particularly associated with CDH with migraine features, rather than with CDH without migraine features. Obesity emerged as a risk factor after adjusting for other comorbidities and demographics. In the study of Scher, CDHs could not have been subclassified as chronic migraine (CM) or chronic tension-type headache (CTTH).

Following the first study, two large epidemiologic studies further investigated the relationship between BMI, episodic migraine and chronic migraine. The first study focused on the relationship between BMI and episodic migraine [13]. A total of 30,215 participants were interviewed, of whom 3791 had migraine. Migraine prevalence, frequency of headache attacks and headache features were modeled as a function of BMI, adjusting by covariates (age, sex, marital status, income, medical treatment, depressive symptoms, medication use). BMI was not associated with the prevalence of migraine. It was, however, associated with the frequency of headache attacks. In the normal weight group, just 4.4% of migraine sufferers had 10–14 headache days per month. This increased to 5.8% of the overweight group [odds ratio (OR) 1.3; 95% confidence interval (CI) = 0.6–2.8], 13.6% of the obese (OR 2.9; 95% CI = 1.9–4.4) and 20.7% of the severely obese (OR 5.7; 95% CI = 3.6–8.8) (Figure 8.1). In adjusted analyses, obesity correlated with frequency of attacks among migraineurs. This study first suggested that although obesity was not a risk factor for migraine, it was associated with increased migraine frequency, and therefore it seemed to be a risk factor for migraine progression.

In the obesity-CDH study, similar methods were used to assess the relationship between BMI and CDH, as well as its subtypes, CM and CTTH [14]. The study confirmed that obesity and CDH are comorbid,

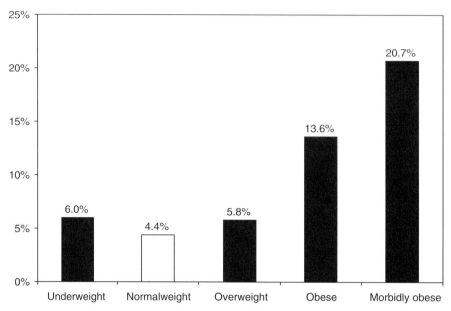

Figure 8.1 Relationship between body mass index and 10–14 days of headache in migraineurs from the population.

after adjusting for several other comorbidities and for demographics. It also suggested that obesity is a much stronger risk factor for CM than for CTTH. For CM, the prevalence ranged from 0.9% in the normal weight group (reference group), to 1.2% of the overweight (OR 1.4; 95% CI = 1.1–1.8), 1.6% of the obese (OR 1.7; 95% CI = 1.2–2.43) and 2.5% of the severely obese (OR 2.2; 95% CI = 1.5–3.2). Underweight subjects (prevalence 1.06%; OR 1.13; 95% CI = 0.6–2.1), did not differ from normal weight. The effects of BMI on the prevalence of CTTH were not significant, except in the severely obese group.

More recently, as a part of the American Migraine Prevalence and Prevention Study (AMPP), a validated questionnaire was mailed to 120,000 households selected to be representative of the US population. Headaches were classified according to the International Headache Society criteria. We identified 18,968 individuals with migraine, 7564 with probable migraine, and 2051 with severe episodic tension-type headache (in the AMPP study, headaches are screened based on the presence of at least one severe headache in the past year). The distribution of very frequent headache (10–14 days/month) was assessed by BMI and headache type. For migraine, contrasted to the normal weight group (6.5% had 10–14 days of headache), the proportion was non-significantly higher in the overweight (7.4%), and higher in the obese (8.2%, $p < 0.001$) and morbidly obese (10.4%, $p < 0.0001$). For probable migraine (PM) and episodic tension-type headache (ETTH), the differences were not significant in the adjusted analyses. The disability of migraineurs, but not

Table 8.1 Summary of the four population studies that investigated the relationship between obesity and migraine progression.

Authors	Comments	Main findings
Scher et al. [12]	• Case control followed by a longitudinal design • Only longitudinal study currently published. • Sample size = 1932	• In the longitudinal arm, the odds of CDH were five times higher in obese and three times higher in overweight subjects, relative to normal weight
Bigal et al. [13]	• Cross-sectional, assessing the influence of obesity on migraine frequency • Sample size = 30,215	• Relative to the normal weight group, the odds of having very frequent headache attacks were 2.9 in the obese and 5.7 in the severely obese
Bigal and Lipton [14]	• Cross-sectional, assessing the relationship between obesity and CDH • Sample size = 30,215	• Chronic daily headache and obesity are associated. Obesity is a stronger risk factor for chronic migraine than for chronic tension-type headache
Bigal et al. [15]	• Cross-sectional, assessing the relationship between obesity and several episodic headaches • Sample size = 30,703 • This study has a longitudinal phase, ongoing	• Obesity was strongly associated with the frequency and severity of the attacks experienced by migraineurs, intermediately associated with probable migraine, and not associated with episodic tension-type headache

CDH, chronic daily headaches.

PM or ETTH sufferers, also varied as a function of BMI. Among migraineurs, 32% of those with normal weight had some disability, vs 37.2% of the overweight ($p < 0.01$), 38.4% of the obese ($p < 0.001$) and 40.9% of the morbidly obese ($p < 0.001$). These findings supported the concept that the obesity is an exacerbating factor for migraine, but not for headaches overall [15].

Table 8.1 summarizes some key points of these four population studies assessing the relationship between headache and migraine progression.

Since obesity is a risk factor for increased migraine attack frequency, and because most of the migraine preventive therapies are not weight neutral, it is of interest to assess whether obesity imposes increased difficulties in the treatment of migraine. Two studies have demonstrated that obesity is not associated with increased refractoriness to preventive or acute migraine therapy [16,17]. However, the risk for cardiovascular disease changes as a function of weight gain secondary to preventive medications. In a study where subjects with migraine were enrolled in a double-blind clinical trial comparing 100 mg/d of topiramate and of amitriptyline, individuals from both treatment groups were pooled and stratified into three groups [18]. The 'major weight gain' group gained ≥5% of their baseline bodyweight at the conclusion of the study; the 'major weight loss' group lost ≥5% of their baseline bodyweight. The third group had a less than 5% weight change. The influence of weight change in headache outcomes, as well as in markers of CVD (blood pressure, C-reactive protein, cholesterol), was assessed using analysis of covariance. Of 331 subjects, 52 (16%) experienced major weight gain, and 56 (17%) experienced major weight loss. Weight change was not associated with differential efficacy for the treatment of headache. However, contrasted with those with major weight loss, those who gained weight experienced elevations in mean diastolic blood pressure (+2.5 vs −1.2 mmHg), heart rate (+7.6 vs −1.3 b.p.m.), glycosylated hemoglobin (+0.09% vs −0.04%), total cholesterol (+6.4 vs −6.3 mg/dL), low-density lipoprotein cholesterol (+7.0 vs −4.4 mg/dL), triglycerides (+15.3 vs −10.4 mg/dL), and an increase in high sensitivity C-reactive protein (+1.8 vs −1.9 mg/L). Both groups experienced decreases in systolic blood pressure (−4.0 vs −1.3 mmHg) and high-density lipoprotein cholesterol (−3.7 vs −0.8 mg/dL). Increased weight during migraine treatment is not associated with poor headache treatment outcomes, but is associated with deterioration of CVD risk markers [2].

Clinical intervention

Although, obesity is now a well-established risk factor for progression, it is unknown if weight loss is related to a decrease in headache frequency. Nonetheless, based on the data, migraineurs should be motivated to maintain their weight (if normal weight) or decrease it (if overweight or obese). This goal requires diets and behavioral support. Orlistat and sibutramine are approved by the US Food and Drug Administration (FDA) for the long-term treatment of obesity [19]. Both low-carbohydrate and low-fat diets promote weight loss.

Since obesity and headache frequency are related, the use of migraine preventive medications that are weight neutral or that are associated with weight loss in those who are overweight or obese may be recommended. Of the FDA-approved migraine medications, only topiramate has been shown to promote weight loss [20]. Beta-blockers and calcium channel blockers are generally weight neutral. Divalproex sodium and tricyclic antidepressants promote weight gain.

Temporomandibular disorders

Among the conditions associated with migraine, temporomandibular disorders (TMD) are rarely mentioned [21,22]. Nonetheless, TMD is of importance for several reasons. First, TMD may be a cause of headache in the disorder referred to as 'headache attributed to TMD', a secondary disorder according to the International Classification of Headache Disorders [23]. Second, TMD may be an exacerbating factor for an independent primary headache disorder [24,25]. Finally, individuals with TMD and primary headaches (e.g. migraine) may experience an added burden because more than one disorder is present (migraine, headache from TMD, other symptoms of TMD).

TMDs are characterized by pain in the muscles of mastication, the temporomandibular joint (TMJ), or both. In addition, signs include tenderness at the temporomandibular joint area, joint sounds (clicks or crepitation), limitations or deviation upon mandibular opening, and 'distance symptoms', such as pain in the neck or headache [26].The gold standard for diagnosing TMD is based on the Research Diagnostic Criteria for TMD (RDC/TMD) [26]. The RDC/TMD criteria, intended for both clinical practice and research, subdivide TMDs into three main groups: TMD due to muscular disorders (Group 1); TMD due to intra-articular disk disorders (Group 2); and mixed TMD (Group 3).

Are TMD and migraine comorbid?

TMD is common in the population. In the USA the overall prevalence of TMD is 4.6% (6.3% for women and 2.8% for men) [27]. Like migraine, TMD is more prevalent in young and middle-aged adults and declines in frequency among the elderly and in women in the postmenopausal years. As for migraine, hormonal factors seem to be of importance in TMD, and the intensity of musculoskeletal pain associated with TMD varies across the menstrual cycle [28].

Limited evidence suggests that migraine and TMD are comorbid. Population-based data suggest that TMD symptoms are more prevalent in individuals with headache than in individuals without headache. Among headache sufferers, TMD symptoms are more common among individuals with migraine and CDH relative to episodic tension-type headache [29]. In a population-based study, 24.5% of subjects who reported headache also reported TMD, while only 13% of subjects without headache experienced TMD [21]. Mitrirattanakul and Merrill also observed that headache prevalence was markedly higher in individuals with TMD (72.7%) than in a control group (31.9%) ($p < 0.001$) [30].

Does TMD influence migraine progression?

While the relevance of TMD for migraine chronification remains unclear, available epidemiologic data suggest a relationship between TMD and primary headache disorders. For example, in a study conducted in Sweden, frequent symptoms of TMD and frequent headache were strongly associated ($p < 0.0001$; OR 4.1; 95% CI = 2.4–6.9) [31]. Similarly, in a large epidemiologic study conducted in Brazil, as contrasted to individuals without TMD, all forms of headache were significantly more common in individuals with TMD. The prevalence ratios (PR) of TMD symptoms were significantly higher in individuals with episodic tension-type headache (ETTH) (PR 1.48; 95% CI = 1.20–1.79), migraine (PR 2.10; 95% CI = 1.80–2.47) and chronic daily headaches (CDH) (PR 2.41; 95% CI = 1.84–3.17) (Figure 8.2). The prevalence of TMD symptoms was very similar in individuals with migraine and CDH and significantly increased in both groups (migraine and CDH) relative to individuals with ETTH. However, a higher number of TMD symptoms (as a metric of TMD

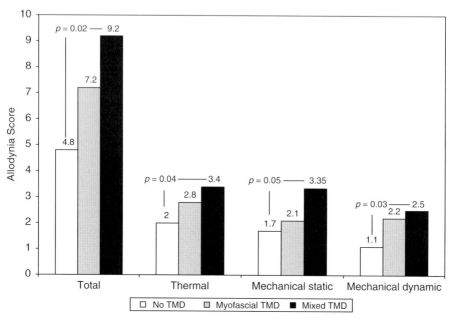

Figure 8.2 Allodynia scores, as measured by the validated ASC-12 questionnaire, as a function of temporomandibular disorder (TMD) status, in migraineurs.

severity) was associated with CDH, suggesting that severity of both, TMD and primary headaches, are correlated [29]. Although a causal relationship cannot be addressed by cross-sectional studies, the link between TMD and frequent headaches was established. Interestingly, a recent study suggested that migraineurs with TMD are more likely to have ictal and interictal allodynia, a know risk factor for chronic migraine [32]. The authors hypothesized that, since neurons in the nucleus caudalis integrate nociceptive input from intracranial and extracranial tissues, and receive supraspinal facilitatory as well as inhibitory inputs, nociceptive inputs from masticatory muscles or the TMJ could lead to activation of the trigeminal nucleus caudalis predisposing to headaches in migraineurs [33].

The treatment of TMD

A detailed discussion of the treatment of TMD is beyond the scope of this chapter. The key message is that doctors should screen for TMD when challenged with refractory migraine patients, or when treating individuals who have progressed to CM without other evident risk factors. The treatment of TMD involves restoring the dynamics of mastication (occlusal surfaces of the teeth and other biodynamic interventions), and other pain-relief measures including analgesics (non-steroidal anti-inflammatory drugs, NSAIDS) and/or off-label use of low-doses of tricyclic antidepressants that have antimuscarinic properties (e.g. amitriptyline, nortriptyline). A careful odontological assessment may be indicated in those suspected of having TMD, and assessment regarding the utility of therapeutic plaques or splints, reconstructive dentistry, orthodontics, arthrocentesis and surgical repositioning of the mandible.

Intranasal contact points

Contact points refer to intranasal contact between opposing mucosal surfaces. Contact points are frequently seen in rhinology clinics, although the prevalence of this anatomic variation in the population is unknown. In a cohort study of 973 patients seen consecutively in a specialty center, contact points were present in 4% of subjects [34].

When contact points are present, headaches may arise as referred pain through the trigeminal system [35]. Therefore, contact points may be a cause of secondary headache or an exacerbating factor for primary headaches [35].

Mucosal contact headache is a newly added secondary headache disorder in the International Classification of Headache Disorders (ICHD-2) [23], supported by limited evidence. According to the ICHD-2, these headaches are characterized by intermittent pain localized in the periorbital and medial canthal or temporozygomatic regions, associated with evidence of mucosal contact points by nasal endoscopy or CT imaging. Acute rhinosinusitis must be excluded. The clinical findings of contact point headaches, according to the ICHD-2 description, correspond to variations in mucosal congestion mediated by gravitational changes. Finally, the ICHD-2 criteria require abolition of headache within 5 minutes following topical application of topical anesthesia to the middle turbinate or contact point area, using placebo or other control, and significant improvement of the headache in less than 7 days after removal of mucosal contact points.

It is unknown whether contact points and migraine are comorbid. We report it in this chapter, however, since limited evidence suggests that, in migraineurs, contact points (as with TMD and obesity) may induce migraine chronification (chronic migraine). This was suggested by a study in which 21 individuals with refractory migraine (to standard migraine therapies) and radiographic evidence of contact points in the sinonasal area were given endoscopic sinus surgery and septoplasty for contact point. To be selected for surgery, patients had to report total abolition of headache pain with intranasal lidocaine. The headache characteristics were assessed preoperatively and at follow-up (6–62 months after surgery) using a standardized questionnaire.

Results were robust, although they should be interpreted with caution, since this was an open, single-center study. Mean headache frequency was reduced from 17.7 to 7.7 headache days per month ($p = 0.003$). Mean headache severity was reduced from 7.8 to 3.6 on a 0–10 scale ($p = 0.0001$). Headache-related disability was reduced from 5.6 (10-point scale) to 1.8 ($p < 0.0001$). A total of 16 subjects (76.2%) had their headache scores improved by 50% or more; nine (42.9%) were pain-free at the last follow-up. A total of 18 (95.8%) had at least a 25% reduction in their headache scores. The headache scores of two patients (9.5%) increased by less than 25% [36–38].

With all the caveats of the data, it may be suggested that for selected patients with refractory headaches, demonstrable contact points, and a positive response to topical decongestant and anesthesia, a surgical approach toward the triggering factor may be useful, pending prospective studies.

References

1 Feinstein AR. The basic elements of clinical science. J Chronic Dis 1963;16:1125–33.
2 Lipton RB, Silberstein SD. Why study the comorbidity of migraine? Neurology 1994;44(10 Suppl. 7):S4–5.
3 Scher AI, Bigal ME, Lipton RB. Comorbidity of migraine. Curr Opin Neurol 2005;18:305–10.
4 Scher AI, Stewart WF, Lipton RB. The comorbidity of headache with other pain syndromes. Headache 2006;46:1416–23.
5 Haut SR, Bigal ME, Lipton RB. Chronic disorders with episodic manifestations: focus on epilepsy and migraine. Lancet Neurol 2006;5:148–57.
6 Kruit MC, van Buchem MA, Hofman PA, et al. Migraine as a risk factor for subclinical brain lesions. JAMA 2004;291:427–34.
7 Kurth T, Slomke MA, Kase CS, et al. Migraine, headache, and the risk of stroke in women: a prospective study. Neurology 2005; 64:1020–6.
8 Kurth T, Gaziano JM, Cook NR, Logroscino G, Diener HC, Buring JE. Migraine and risk of cardiovascular disease in women. JAMA 2006;296:283–91.
9 Tietjen GE, Peterlin BL, Brandes JL, et al. Depression and anxiety: effect on the migraine-obesity relationship. Headache 2007;47:866–75.
10 Gilbert GJ. Obesity and migraine: a population study. Neurology 2007;68:241; author reply 241.
11 Iwasaki Y, Ikeda K. Obesity and migraine: a population study. Neurology 2007;68:241; author reply 241.
12 Scher AI, Stewart WF, Ricci JA, Lipton RB. Factors associated with the onset and remission of chronic daily headache in a population-based study. Pain 2003;106:81–9.
13 Bigal ME, Liberman JN, Lipton RB. Obesity and migraine: a population study. Neurology 2006;66:545–50.
14 Bigal ME, Lipton RB. Obesity is a risk factor for transformed migraine but not chronic tension-type headache. Neurology 2006;67:252–7.
15 Bigal ME, Tsang A, Loder E, Serrano D, Reed ML, Lipton RB. Body mass index and episodic headaches: a population-based study. Arch Intern Med 2007;167:1964–70.
16 Bigal ME, Gironda M, Tepper SJ, et al. Headache prevention outcome and body mass index. Cephalalgia 2006;26:445–50.
17 Bigal ME, Lipton RB, Biondi D, Xiand J, Hulihan J. Weight change and clinical markers of cardiovascular disease risk during preventive treatment of migraine. Cephalalgia. 2009 Nov;29(11):1188–96.
18 Dodick DW, Freitag F, Banks J, et al., for the CAPSS-277 Investigator Group. Topiramate versus amitriptyline in migraine prevention: a 26-week, multicenter, randomized, double-blind, parallel-group noninferiority trial in adult migraineurs. Clin Ther. 2009 Mar;31(3):542–59.

19 Sidhaye A, Cheskin LJ. Pharmacologic treatment of obesity. Adv Psychosom Med 2006;27:42–52.

20 Silberstein SD, Hulihan J, Karim MR, et al. Efficacy and tolerability of topiramate 200 mg/d in the prevention of migraine with/without aura in adults: a randomized, placebo-controlled, double-blind, 12-week pilot study. Clin Ther 2006;28:1002–11.

21 Ciancaglini R, Radaelli G. The relationship between headache and symptoms of temporomandibular disorder in the general population. J Dent 2001;29:93–8.

22 De Kanter RJ, Truin GJ, Burgersdijk RC, et al. Prevalence in the Dutch adult population and a meta-analysis of signs and symptoms of temporomandibular disorder. J Dent Res 1993;72:1509–18.

23 Classification Committee of the International Headache Society. The International Classification of Headache Disorders, 2nd edition. Cephalalgia 2004;24(Suppl. 1):1–149.

24 Lupoli TA, Lockey RF. Temporomandibular dysfunction: an often overlooked cause of chronic headaches. Ann Allergy Asthma Immunol 2007;99:314–18.

25 Magnusson T, Carlsson GE. Recurrent headaches in relation to temporomandibular joint pain-dysfunction. Acta Odontol Scand 1978;36:333–8.

26 Dworkin SF, LeResche L. Research diagnostic criteria for temporomandibular disorders: review, criteria, examinations and specifications, critique. J Craniomandib Disord 1992;6:301–55.

27 Isong U, Gansky SA, Plesh O. Temporomandibular joint and muscle disorder-type pain in U.S. adults: the National Health Interview Survey. J Orofac Pain 2008;22:317–22.

28 LeResche L. Epidemiology of temporomandibular disorders: implications for the investigation of etiologic factors. Crit Rev Oral Biol Med 1997;8:291–305.

29 Gonçalves AD, Speciali JG, Jales L, Camparis C, Bigal ME. Temporo-mandibular symptoms, migraine and chronic daily headaches in the population. Neurology. 2009 Aug 25;73(8):645–6.

30 Mitrirattanakul S, Merrill RL. Headache impact in patients with orofacial pain. J Am Dent Assoc 2006;137:1267–74.

31 Storm C, Wanman A. A two-year follow-up study of temporomandibular disorders in a female Sami population: validation of cases and controls as predicted by questionnaire. Acta Odontol Scand 2007;65:341–7.

32 Bigal ME, Ashina S, Burstein R, et al. Prevalence and characteristics of allodynia in headache sufferers: a population study. Neurology 2008;70:1525–33.

33 Bevilacqua-Grossi D, Grosberg B, Napchan U, Lipton R, Bigal ME. Temporomandibular disorders and cutaneous allodynia are associated in individuals with migraine. Cephalalgia. 2010 Apr; 30(4):425–32.

34 Abu-Bakra M, Jones NS. Prevalence of nasal mucosal contact points in patients with facial pain compared with patients without facial pain. J Laryngol Otol 2001;115:629–32.

35 Tosun F, Gerek M, Ozkaptan Y. Nasal surgery for contact point headaches. Headache 2000;40:237–40.

36 Behin F, Lipton RB, Bigal M. Migraine and intranasal contact point headache: is there any connection? Curr Pain Headache Rep 2006;10:312–15.

37 Behin F, Behin B, Bigal ME, Lipton RB. Surgical treatment of patients with refractory migraine headaches and intranasal contact points. Cephalalgia 2005;25:439–43.

38 Behin F, Behin B, Behin D, Baredes S. Surgical management of contact point headaches. Headache 2005;45:204–10.

9 Migraine Comorbidities in Children

Çiçek Wöber-Bingöl[1] and Andrew Hershey[2]

[1] Department of Psychiatry of Childhood and Adolescence, Medical University of Vienna, Vienna, Austria

[2] Department of Pediatrics, Division of Neurology, Cincinnati Children's Hospital Medical Center and University of Cincinnati College of Medicine, Cincinnati, OH, USA

Introduction

Managing headache in young patients requires a comprehensive view of the problem, not focusing on headache itself but also considering comorbidity, psychosocial aspects and the patients' environments [1]. In this chapter, we will summarize the scientific evidence and we will illustrate the scope of the problem with a few case reports.

'Comorbidity' is a general medical term that dates back to Feinsten. The current conceptualization of the term implies an association, more than casual, but probably not causal, between an index disease and one, or more, coexisting physical or psychiatric disorders [2].

The identification of medical and psychiatric comorbidities has just begun in children and adolescents. However, the degree to which these comorbidities influence the expression and outcome of pediatric headache remains uncertain. Part of the difficulty in identifying comorbidities is separating out comorbidities from secondary headaches. One potential way of differentiating these is to limit the study of the potential secondary conditions to only those patients who have an underlying primary headache disorder. For the purposes of this review, this will be further limited to only patients with migraine.

The epidemiology of these comorbidities in pediatric and adolescent migraine patients is largely unknown. The majority of the reports on comorbidities are based on observations within headache specialty practices, and thus have a referral bias. They do provide an estimate of these conditions in patients with frequent or disabling headaches.

The pathophysiology of these comorbidities should be expected to be similar to adults with the same conditions. For many of these conditions this exact interrelationship is not known and may be due to a general biological stressor that can be broadly applied, while others may have a more defined etiology.

Asthma and allergic disorders

Asthma and related allergic disorders including sinusitis are a common problem in children and adolescents. Approximately, 9% of children and adolescents have asthma, and this increases to 32% for any allergic condition [3]. Given this high prevalence, it is not surprising that many patients with migraine also have allergic symptoms. This overlap often creates confusion in the underlying diagnosis, and in adults has led to the misdiagnosis of sinusitis or allergic rhinitis for migraine [4].

Migraine itself has a neuroinflammatory component, and it could be expected that in patients with immunologic or inflammatory conditions there may be an increased risk of migraine. In an allergy-based clinical evaluation, 45.9% of the children being seen for allergy independently reported having recurrent headaches, the majority of which meet International Classification of Headache Disorders, second edition (ICHD-2), criteria for migraine [5]. The underlying etiology may be due to an inflammatory disorder, or due to the stress of two chronic conditions and therefore be a generic comorbid response.

For young children, cyproheptadine has been used for migraine prevention and may have a benefit for treating allergies. It can be limiting for older children due to the side effects of increased appetite and lethargy. The use of leukotriene inhibitors has been tried for a small group of children, and shown benefit in an uncontrolled study. A larger concern, however, should be the avoidance of beta-blockers in these patients as they may exacerbate exercise-induced asthma. In addition, if the patient has nasal polyps and asthma, they may be at risk of aspirin (non-steroidal anti-inflammatory drugs, NSAID) sensitivity and have an exacerbation of their asthma symptoms if treated with NSAIDs for their migraine.

Cardiovascular disease

In adults there may be a relationship between cardiovascular disease and migraine. This has not been well described in children. As many of the cardiovascular syndromes in children are due to congenital heart defects, there may be a degree of compensation by the time the patients begin to express their migraine.

The correlation between migraine and patent foramen ovale (PFO) is still debatable. Initial studies indicated an increased prevalence of PFO in migraineurs with aura, and an increased prevalence of migraine and migraine with aura in persons with PFO. Initial retrospective analyses of PFO closure suggest clinically significant improvements in migraine patterns. Schwedt et al. [6] reviewed data correlating migraine and PFO. Their aims were to examine the prevalence of migraine in patients with PFO, the prevalence of PFO in migraineurs, and the effect of PFO closure on migraine. They conducted a quantitative systematic review of articles on migraine and PFO that met inclusion criteria, then reviewed, appraised and subjected the articles to data extraction. Of 134 articles identified, 18 met *a priori* selection criteria. The estimated strength of association between PFO and migraine, reflected by summary odds ratios (ORs), was 5.13 [95% confidence interval (CI) = 4.67–5.59], and between PFO and migraine with aura the OR was 3.21 (95% CI = 2.38–4.17). The grade of evidence was low. The association between migraine and PFO was OR 2.54 (95% CI = 2.01–3.08). The grade of evidence was low to moderate. Six studies of PFO closure suggested improvement in migraine, but had a very low grade of evidence. The low-to-moderate grade of evidence from observational studies supports an apparent association between PFO and migraine. Although PFO closure seemed to affect migraine patterns favorably, the very low grade of available evidence to support this association precludes definitive conclusions.

Stroke

An increased risk for stroke in teenage girls and young women with probable migraine with aura has been noticed, particularly for those who smoke or use oral contraceptives, compared with women who do not have migraines. Kittner and colleagues assessed the link between probable migraine with visual aura (PMVA) and probable migraine without visual aura with ischemic stroke among groups of women [7]. Using data from a population-based, case-control study, they studied 386 women aged 15 to 49 years with first ischemic stroke and 614 age- and ethnicity-matched controls. Based on their responses to a questionnaire on headache symptoms, subjects were classified as having no migraine, probable migraine without visual aura, or probable migraine with visual aura (PMVA) according to various factors including headache characteristics and various clinical features. The results showed that young women with PMVA had 1.5 greater odds of ischemic stroke (95% CI = 1.1–2.0); the risk was highest in those with no history of hypertension, diabetes or myocardial infarction compared to women with no migraine. Women with PMVA who were current cigarette smokers and current users of oral contraceptives had 7.0-fold higher odds of stroke (95% CI = 1.3–22.8) than did women with PMVA who were non-smokers and not users of oral contraceptives. Women with onset of PMVA within the previous year had 6.9-fold higher adjusted odds of stroke (95% CI = 2.3–21.2) compared to women with no history of migraine. Their conclusion was that PMVA was associated with an increased risk of stroke, particularly among young women and teenage girls without other medical conditions associated with stroke. Behavioral risk factors, specifically smoking and oral contraceptive use, markedly increased the risk of PMVA, as did recent onset of PMVA. PMVA may be a risk factor for stroke or these patients may be genetically predisposed for both, with the migraine or the stroke being a comorbidity.

Epilepsy

In studies of pediatric epilepsy patients it has been observed that a larger than expected proportion of these patients and their families have a history of migraine. This relationship appeared to be even higher for children who had migraine with aura [8]. The recognition of migraine and epilepsy as comorbid requires the separation of post-ictal headaches as these are more of a direct triggering of the headache by the seizure.

In patients who have both migraine and epilepsy, antiepileptic therapy should be the primary preventive focus. Although no antiepileptic drugs (AEDs) have been approved for the prevention of pediatric and adolescent migraine, several of the agents used in adult migraineurs have been demonstrated to be safe and effective in the treatment of pediatric epilepsy. These include divalproate, topiramate and gabapentin, as well as, potentially, newer agents such as levetiracetam, zonisamide and pregabalin. The choice of AED should be guided by the underlying epilepsy syndrome, but should include a medication with prospective migraine preventive properties. The goals of treatment vary; for migraine the aim is one to two headaches per month for 4 to 6 months, whereas for epilepsy the goal is seizure freedom for 2 years. Thus the epilepsy treatment dictates the duration of AED use.

Obesity

Obesity is an area of growing concern in children and adolescents. Worldwide the incidence of obesity in childhood and adolescence is increasing. In adults there may be a direct contribution of obesity to headache frequency. In obese children and children at risk of becoming obese there is an effect on both headache frequency and disability – based on a body mass index (BMI) above the 85th percentile [9]. This needs to be addressed in the overall treatment plan, as it appears that those children who can lower their BMI percentile have a greater improvement than those who don't lose weight. Furthermore, those who continue to gain weight may actually have a worsening of both their headache frequency and disability.

Sleep disorders

Disturbances in sleep can have both a biological and a behavioral basis. Sleep deprivation is one of the most common triggers of migraine in children and adolescents. This is complicated by the biological changes affecting sleep that occur during puberty, causing adolescents to have delayed sleep onset, which is hormonally controlled, in conflict with many school systems that require these children to wake earlier than is biologically natural.

In addition, there may be specific sleep disturbances in children [10] and adolescents [11]. In children (aged 2–12) more sleep disturbances were seen in children with migraine, with a correlation between both frequency and duration of headache attacks and sleep anxiety, parasomnias and bedtime resistance. In adolescents, the sleep disturbances were commonly related to sleep behaviorisms, including 65.7% having inadequate sleep; contributory factors were found to include difficulty falling asleep (40.6%) and night wakings (38%), resulting in 23.3% with daytime sleepiness.

Sleep management therefore becomes an essential part in both the evaluation of these issues as well as in management to overcome these disruptions.

Learning disabilities

The term learning disabilities (LD) comprises difficulties in a broad range of academic and functional skills such as listening, speaking, reading, writing, reasoning, mathematics, coordination, spatial adaptation and memorization. These difficulties can occur alone or in varying combinations, and can range from mild to severe.

The causes of LD are not well understood, and sometimes there is no apparent cause. In some cases LD are related to heredity, problems during pregnancy and birth, head injuries, malnutrition, or toxic exposure, behavioral or social factors.

By using data from the National Survey of Children's Health, the overall lifetime prevalence of LD in US children in 2003 was calculated to be 9.7% (95% CI = 9.4–10.1), meaning that an estimated 6 million US children aged below 18 years had LD at some stage in their life [12]. From experience in a tertiary headache center, LD are more frequently seen in children with migraine. In an epidemiologic study, LD were more frequently reported in children with frequent or severe headaches (OR 1.59; 95% CI = 1.26–2.02) [13]. Although LD are considered to be lifelong disorders, academic skills themselves can be improved with targeted interventions. Practice is a particularly important component in developing competence. Specialized instructions are designed to make improvements in the weak areas. In addition, adjustments and equipment such as electronic dictionaries or word spellers are intended to accommodate or help compensate for the disabilities. In children with migraine experiencing a significant increase in attack frequency after school entry, LD should be considered as an underlying cause, even though evidence from controlled trials is lacking.

Attention deficit hyperactivity disorder

Attention deficit hyperactivity disorder (ADHD) is the most common psychiatric disorder in children. Eight to twelve percent of children are affected worldwide. The onset is before 7 years of age. ADHD is

characterized by a persistent pattern of inattention, hyperactivity and
impulsiveness. At least half of children with the disorder will have
impairing symptoms in adulthood. Twin, adoption and molecular
genetic studies show ADHD to be highly heritable, and other findings
have recorded obstetric complications and psychosocial adversity as
predisposing risk factors [14]. Little is known about the association
between migraine and ADHD. In an epidemiologic study [13] including
subjects aged 4–18 years, the prevalence of attention deficit disorder was
significantly higher in individuals with frequent or severe headache (OR
2.02; 95% CI = 1.56–2.64).

Gilles de la Tourette syndrome

Tourette syndrome (TS) is one of the most common childhood genetic
movement disorders, with a reported frequency in children as high as 3%.
The condition is characterized by motor and phonic tics that fluctuate in
distribution, severity and frequency. TS is associated with attention deficit
with or without hyperactivity, obsessive-compulsive traits, and other
neurobehavioral comorbidities, such as poor impulse control, self
injurious behavior, anxiety and mood disorders. The frequency of
migraine headache in a clinic sample of TS subjects including 62 children
and 38 adults was nearly four-fold more than the frequency of migraines
reported in the general population [15].

Depression

Depression is a common disorder in children and adolescents. A lifetime
prevalence of serious depression is found in approximately 5% of subjects
younger than 18 years of age. The prevalence of depression increases with
age, especially after the onset of puberty. There is no gender-related
difference in children. Onset of puberty, however, is associated with a
marked increase in the rate of depression among females, with a female to
male ratio of 2:1. The prevalence of depression may be higher in children
with other psychiatric disorders, such as ADHD or anxiety disorders, and in
those with general medical conditions such as diabetes, asthma or cancer.

   The comorbidity of migraine and depression has been investigated
frequently and carefully in adults [16]. In contrast, there is far less evidence
in children and adolescents. In 2008, Amouroux and Rousseau-Salvador
[17] reviewed studies on the relation between migraine, anxiety and
depression, and selected those specifying the diagnostic criteria of migraine
and using validated measures for anxiety and depression. Of 11 articles,
10 used a control group matched for age and sex. Only three of the studies
used a representative sample of the general population. The studies
included do not provide conclusive findings for the comorbidity of
migraine, anxiety and depression in children. The majority of the studies
with clinical populations show slightly higher scores on at least one of the

anxiety or depression scales in the migraine group as compared to the control group. However, in all 11 studies, the average score on the anxiety and depression scales in children with migraine did not reach a pathological level, according to the norms established by the validated scales. Findings point to above-average levels of anxiety or depression, rather than diagnosed psychopathologies. None of the three studies carried out in the general population revealed differences between the anxiety and depression scores in children with migraine as opposed to children in the control group. The difference in results from studies in the general population and clinical populations can most likely be explained by a recruitment bias.

In a longitudinal epidemiologic study on 'functionally impairing headache', Pine et al. [18] found headache to be twice as common in depressed adolescents than in non-depressed adolescents. Major depression in adolescents, without current or past headache, prospectively predicted the new onset of headaches in young adulthood. Among adolescents without a history of chronic impairing headache, those with current major depression face a nearly ten-fold increased risk of developing such headaches at some time during the next 7 years.

Studying the relationship between migraine and suicidal ideation in a non-referred sample of adolescents, Wang et al. [19] found that suicidal ideation was reported more frequently by subjects with migraine compared to non-migraine subjects (16.1% vs 6.2%; OR 2.9; 95% CI = 2.3–3.6; $p = 0.001$). After controlling for depression score and sociodemographic characteristics, the association remained for migraine with aura (adjusted OR 1.79; 95% CI = 1.07–2.99; $p = 0.025$) and high headache frequency (>7 days/month; adjusted OR 1.69; 95% CI = 1.12–2.56; $p = 0.013$) but not for migraine without aura or probable migraine.

Anxiety disorders

Anxiety disorders comprise generalized anxiety disorder, panic disorder, phobias, obsessive-compulsive disorder, post-traumatic stress disorder and separation anxiety.

Children with migraine lose more school days than healthy children. Many children who present with school fear or school phobia may actually have a history of primary headache [20]. The presence of a comorbid psychiatric condition tends to worsen the course of primary headaches by increasing the frequency and severity of attacks, thus making the headache less responsive to treatment and increasing the risk of chronification [20]. It is also likely that children who have school phobia and migraine tend to get more migraine attacks, which result in a long school absence. Migraine and school phobia might aggravate each other causing an increasing number of days of absence from school.

In a clinic-based follow-up study, Guidetti et al. [21] assessed the relation between migraine, tension-type headache and various psychiatric disorders including anxiety disorders, sleep disorders, adjustment disorder, elimination disorders, eating disorders, mood disorders and school disorders. Generalized anxiety disorder was the most frequent psychiatric diagnosis, and anxiety disorder at baseline was related to enduring headache and migraine. Merikangas et al. [22] postulated a so-called 'syndromic relationship' between migraine and psychiatric disorders on the grounds of their findings. According to this 'syndromic relationship' the first manifestation of migraine is preceded by the occurrence of anxiety disorders in childhood and adolescence, whereas the first manifestation of depression succeeds the first manifestation of migraine. In contrast, studies in the general population reviewed by Amouroux and Rousseau-Salvador [17], did not show a relation between migraine and anxiety disorder. As mentioned above the discrepancy between population-based and clinic-based studies is most probably due to selection bias, since patients presenting to a headache center may be more severely affected. Population-based studies increase our knowledge about general aspects of a disease. Clinic-based studies, however, may be more relevant for daily practice, since they reflect the characteristics of those patients actually presenting to a physician.

Case reports

The following unpublished cases from the headache outpatient clinic of the Department of Psychiatry of Childhood and Adolescence at the Medical University of Vienna show that undiscovered medical, psychiatric or psychosocial problems may have an impact on the course of migraine.

Case 1

An underlying disease, which has not been discovered yet, may cause an increase in migraine frequency. A 15-year-old boy experienced an increase in migraine frequency parallel to newly developed right shoulder pain. None of the doctors consulted had a look at the boy's shoulder or examined the painful region. Some gave NSAIDs, others prescribed migraine prophylaxis. At presentation to the headache outpatient clinic a large tumor in the right upper arm was seen and diagnostic work-up revealed non-Hodgkin lymphoma. After months of treatment inducing complete remission, migraine frequency began to decrease significantly.

Case 2

A young girl suffering from frequent migraine attacks and being absent from school on numerous days was prescribed various prophylactic medications by several physicians, but migraine did not improve. At referral to the headache outpatient clinic of the Department of Psychiatry of Childhood and Adolescence, a thorough history-taking revealed the following family background. The parents loved each other. The wife became pregnant in her late 30s, and the couple were very happy with their healthy girl. At the age of 2 years the girl suffered from a severe infection, which led the parents to resume taking the child to their own bedroom (after she had started to sleep in her own room). Some time later the mother got sick and subsequently developed anxiety disorder. The growing girl needed more space in the bed and therefore the loving father began to sleep in the child's room. The parents were focused on preventing their daughter from getting a severe infection and on dealing with the mother's anxiety disorder. The patient did not sleep in her own bedroom until she presented to the headache outpatient clinic at between 14 and 15 years of age. She had developed frequent severe attacks of migraine without aura and started not going to school. She had been successful at school and she was sad about missing school. Nevertheless, she avoided school and stayed alone at home while the parents were at work. The girl was seen by different doctors. She was treated with beta-blockers, dihydroergotamine and antidepressants without any effect. The condition at home became more and more difficult, an atmosphere of fear and anxiety arose, and the girl was finally brought to the headache outpatient clinic. The problems of symbiosis and anxiety disorder were openly explained to the family. A therapeutic setting was established and the first aim was that the girl should start to sleep in her own room again. Initially, the girl experienced a series of severe migraine attacks and it took her 3 weeks to spend all night in her own room, but managing this first step was the beginning of the success. Therapy comprised relaxation training, keeping a success diary and parents' education. After 6 months the headache frequency had decreased to two per month, the girl was successful at school again and she had developed interests appropriate to her age, spending time with her peer group. This example demonstrates that comorbidity of migraine is not unidirectional, and may include the whole family structure; it emphasizes that it is essential to pay attention to the patient's environment.

Case 3

An 8-year-old girl was one of three children of a divorced woman who experienced chronic stress at her work place. The child was brought to the headache outpatient clinic having four migraine attacks per week. The face of the girl was a suffering face. The mother had no relatives in the city. The girl's father called only twice a year and the children did not even know where he lived. He sent maintenance irregularly. The family had not had a real holiday for several years. The mother worked up to 4.00 pm five days a week. She had nobody who could spend some time with her children. All children attended school. After work the mother picked up the children from school and spent her time with them until she took them to bed. Thereafter, she did the housework, sometimes until 2 a.m. In the morning, it was very hard for the mother to wake up on time. Usually, the children had to leave without breakfast 15 minutes after getting up. The morning was full of hurry and stress. The patient – the only one of the three children suffering from migraine – developed more and more attacks and she was extremely afraid of the next attack. In the light of all her problems, the child was admitted for inpatient treatment. The child underwent biofeedback and learned a more regular lifestyle. The mother also got support. Finally, multidisciplinary management achieved a marked change in the life(style) of the family and a substantial decrease in the girl's migraine attacks.

References

1 Wöber-Bingöl Ç. What does it mean to treat headache in children and adolescents? Dealing with patients; dealing with parents; dealing with teachers. In: Guidetti V, Russell G, Sillanpää M, Winner P (eds) Headache and Migraine in Childhood and Adolescence. London: Martin Dunitz, 2002; 459–66.

2 Galli F, Guidetti V. Psychiatric co-morbidity. In: Guidetti V, Russell G, Sillanpää M, Winner P (eds) Headache and Migraine in Childhood and Adolescence. London: Martin Dunitz, 2002; 181–94.

3 Bloom B, Cohen RA, Freeman G. Summary health statistics for U.S. children: National Health Interview Survey, 2007. Vital Health Statistics 10. 2009 Jan(239):1–80.

4 Cady RK, Schreiber CP. Sinus headache: a clinical conundrum. Otolaryngol Clin North Am 2004;37:267–88.

5 Khurana Hershey G, Stevenson M, Grube E, Hershey A. Characterization of headache presenting to a tertiary allergy clinic. Cephalalgia 2005;25:1004.

6 Schwedt TJ, Demaerschalk BM, Dodick DW. Patent foramen ovale and migraine: a quantitative systematic review. Cephalalgia 2008;28:531–40.

7 MacClellan LR, Giles W, Cole J, et al. Probable migraine with visual aura and risk of ischemic stroke. The Stroke Prevention in Young Women Study. Stroke 2007;38:2438–45.

8 Piccinelli P, Borgatti R, Nicoli F, et al. Relationship between migraine and epilepsy in pediatric age. Headache 2006;46:413–21.

9 Hershey AD, Powers SW, Nelson TD, et al. Obesity in the pediatric headache population: a multicenter study. Headache 2009;49:170–7.

10 Miller VA, Palermo TM, Powers SW, Scher MS, Hershey AD. Migraine headaches and sleep disturbances in children. Headache 2003; 43:362–8.

11 Gilman DK, Palermo TM, Kabbouche MA, Hershey AD, Powers SW. Primary headache and sleep disturbances in adolescents. Headache 2007;47:1189–94.

12 Altarac M, Saroha E. Lifetime prevalence of learning disability among US children. Pediatrics 2007;119(Suppl. 1):S77–83.

13 Lateef TM, Merikangas KR, He J, et al. Headache in a national sample of American children: prevalence and comorbidity. J Child Neurol 2009;24:536–43.

14 Biederman J, Faraone SV. Attention-deficit hyperactivity disorder. Lancet 2005;366:237–48.

15 Kwak C, Vuong KD, Jankovic J. Migraine headache in patients with Tourette syndrome. Arch Neurol 2003;60:1595–8.

16 Hamelsky SW, Lipton RB. Psychiatric comorbidity of migraine. Headache 2006;46:1327–33.

17 Amouroux R, Rousseau-Salvador C. Anxiety and depression in children and adolescents with migraine: a review of the literature. Encephale 2008;34:504–10.

18 Pine DS, Cohen P, Brook J. The association between major depression and headache: results of a longitudinal epidemiologic study in youth. J Child Adolesc Psychopharmacol 1996;6:153–64.

19 Wang SJ, Fuh JL, Juang KD, Lu SR. Migraine and suicidal ideation in adolescents aged 13 to 15 years. Neurology 2009;72:1146–52.

20 Oelkers-Ax R, Resch F. Headache in children and psychiatric problems. Psychiatric Times 2004;11:8–9.

21 Guidetti V, Galli F, Fabrizi P, et al. Headache and psychiatric comorbidity: clinical aspects and outcome in an 8-year follow-up study. Cephalalgia 1998;18:455–62.

22 Merikangas KR, Angst J, Isler H. Migraine and psychopathology. Arch Gen Psychiatry 1990;47:849–53.

10 Optimal Management of Migraine Taking into Account Comorbidities and 'Positive Side Effects'

Peter S. Sándor[1], David W. Dodick[2] and Jean Schoenen[3]

[1] Department of Neurology, Canton Hospital Baden & Rehaclinic Zurzach, Baden Dätwill, Switzerland
[2] Department of Neurology, Mayo Clinic Arizona, Phoenix, AZ, USA
[3] Headache Research Unit, Department of Neurology, Citadelle Hospital, Liège, Belgium

Preventive therapy of migraine

Preventive therapy of migraine has the purpose of diminishing the probability and frequency of attacks. Preventive treatments may also reduce the duration and severity of acute attacks, and in the experience of the authors, preventive therapy may render acute attacks more responsive to acute therapies. This is in contrast to the effect of acute medications, such as triptans and ergots, which are used in the context of acute migraine attacks and tend to increase, rather than decrease, the probability of migraine attacks (medication overuse headache), especially when taken on a regular basis on more than 10 days per months. In contrast to acute medications, preventive medications are intended to be used daily to obtain the best results; see reviews by Silberstein and Goadsby (2002) [1], and Dodick and Silberstein (2007) [2].

Disorders and comorbidities

In a given context, which health problem is considered the main problem and which a comorbid disorder depends on the medical context and the specialty of the treating physician.

Two disorders are defined as comorbid if the second disorder is more prevalent in patients suffering from the first disorder than in a control population, and vice versa. Which of the two is defined as the 'first' disorder often depends on the impact on the patient's life, and the resulting medical context, but it can be completely arbitrary and depend on the treating physician's viewpoint. For instance, in a patient with migraine, obesity and a bipolar disorder, a neurologist, an internist, and a psychiatrist might have different opinions on the most important health problem.

Different types of therapeutic effects and side effects

Pharmacological agents may have different types of effects in the same patient at one point in time or, if various pathologies occur in sequence, at different time points. Based on the above considerations concerning 'main disorder' and comorbidities, it depends on the medical context of therapy which of several pharmacological effects is considered the main effect, and which one the treatment of a comorbidity.

The therapeutic relationship between migraine and its comorbidities depends on the causal link between the disorders. In most instances, this causal link is not completely understood and there is rarely one single treatment providing optimal improvement for both migraine and the

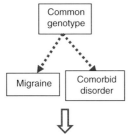

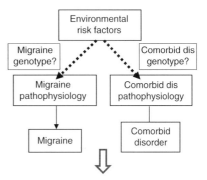

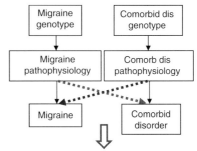

Figure 10.1 The four possible models of causal relationships between migraine and a comorbid disorder and implications for present and future therapy.

comorbid disorder. Future research will, however, improve knowledge on the pathogenetic link between migraine and comorbidities, and thus create opportunities for targeted therapies. Figure 10.1 gives an overview of possible therapeutic strategies depending on the model of the causal relationship between migraine and the comorbid disorder.

In addition to the foregoing, there is a third category of effects in pharmacotherapy, called 'side effects'. Such effects are supposed to be of no utility for the treatment of migraine, but in most cases they influence the patients' well-being or have other medical implications, for instance in the context of pharmacological interactions. Some side effects clearly have a beneficial effect on comorbid disorders and can thus be used as therapeutic effects for these disorders.

If, for instance, in the above mentioned patient with migraine, obesity and bipolar disorder, topiramate is prescribed and causes fatigue as a side effect, in a neurologist's practice the antimigraine effect will be considered as the main therapeutic effect, weight loss and the mood-stabilizing effect as treatment of comorbidities, and fatigue as a negative side effect.

'Positive' side effects

For most patients, side effects have negative and often frightening implications. Negative side effects tend to diminish patients' compliance, as they tend to be unpleasant and therefore decrease patients' motivation for regular medication intake. However, depending on the therapeutic context and also the mode of application, side effects can be rendered positive, without actually treating comorbidities.

In our index patient, suffering from migraine, obesity, and bipolar disorder and taking topiramate, the side effect of fatigue could be negative and interfere with daily activities in a negative way. On the other hand, it could be the case that this patient suffers from some mild insomnia, not severe enough to be considered as clearly pathological, but nevertheless causing some degree of discomfort as she is not always able to fall asleep fast enough and sometimes starts to worry about the slight sleeping problem. If in this female patient, for whom dosing would be 75 mg per day (25–0–50 mg), it might be the case that the fatigue caused by the 50 mg bedtime dose sufficiently influences sleep onset to prevent the patient from worrying. This side effect would thus have a significantly positive impact on her quality of life – in addition to the above mentioned therapeutic effects, and in this case fatigue could be considered a positive side effect.

To be able to take advantage of positive side effects of medications, rather extensive information from the patient is needed. Most often, some degree of 'fine-tuning' is necessary in the therapeutic process as well. This requires significant education and monitoring on the part of both physician and patient. Patients must understand the usual side effects from certain medications and, importantly, the fact that many are temporary and diminish or disappear with time. Inadequate patient education and unrealistic expectations invariably lead to poor patient compliance, lapse from therapy, and suboptimal outcomes. Positive side effects certainly strengthen the motivation of the patient for better compliance. In clinical practice, in patients who are not obese but have a body mass index at the upper normal limit and would like to lose some weight, topiramate is often preferred in spite of its potential for some clearly negative side effects such as cognitive impairment.

Selecting preventive migraine medications based on the presence of comorbid disorders

Since all preventive therapies used for migraine have been developed and initially approved for other indications, these medications not surprisingly have effects on other disorders, many of which may be comorbid with migraine (e.g. epilepsy, depression). As comprehensively demonstrated in this book, a number of disorders are comorbid with migraine and have an actual or potential impact on the patients' health and well-being, and potentially on the clinical course of migraine itself.

Table 10.1 gives an overview over various preventive substances used in migraine, according to effects on the comorbidities discussed in this book. Recommended dosages and the most important side effects and contraindications are also given in Table 10.1. Assuming the diagnosis of migraine has been established and comorbid conditions recognized, this table could serve as a practical guide for clinicians.

Some of the substances can be used against several different comorbidities at the same time, such as beta-blockers, which have an antihypertensive as well as an anxiolytic effect. Antiepileptic drugs can, in general, be used in comorbid pain conditions, such as neuropathic pain, and, of course, also in comorbid epilepsy, which compared to comorbid pain disorders is relatively rare. ACE (angiotensin-converting enzyme) inhibitors and sartans have an antihypertensive effect and can be used in patients suffering from a variety of heart conditions. Antidepressants, being effective against depression and anxiety, are often also useful in the treatment of neuropathic pain and insomnia. Furthermore, there is the group of metabolic enhancers, such as riboflavin, coenzyme Q10 and possibly also magnesium, that can be used in the absence of comorbidities, and have the characteristic of being well tolerated, which makes them a treatment of choice for some clinicians, when combination therapies with the other mentioned classes of substances are planned.

In clinical practice, it happens frequently that a patient already has a treatment for a disorder comorbid with migraine. For optimal management, adequate communication between medical specialists is necessary in order to coordinate the respective pharmacotherapies [3].

As shown schematically in Table 10.2, three situations can occur regarding the reciprocal influence of migraine and comorbidity therapies: neutral, positive/beneficial, and negative/deleterious. In the ideal situation (Table 10.2, first line, first column – 'green light'), the antimigraine preventive treatment has a strong beneficial effect on the comorbid

Table 10.1 Synopsis of the most important evidence-based migraine preventive substances, focusing on comorbidity. Dosages as well as the most important side effects and contraindications are shown.

Comorbidities, special circumstances	Group	Substance	Dosage	Side effects	Contraindications
Arterial hypertension, anxiety without depression	Beta-blocker	Propranolol Metoprolol Bisoprolol (Nadolol) Atenolol Timolol	Individual (as large as possible w/o side effects)	Depression, fatigue, dizziness, sleep disturbances, impotence	Asthma, congestive heart failure, Raynaud's
Epilepsy, neuropathic pain	Antiepileptic drug	Valproate	500–1500 mg/d	Dizziness, tremor, hair loss, hirsutism, teratogenicity, ± fatigue	Pregnancy, hepatitis
Neuropathic pain, epilepsy	Antiepileptic drug	Gabapentin	900–3600 mg/d	Dizziness, drowsiness, fatigue, weight gain	Renal failure
Arterial hypertension	ACE inhibitor	Lisinopril	20 mg/d	Cough, dizziness	Pregnancy (second and third trimesters)
Arterial hypertension	ACE inhibitor	Candesartan	16 mg/d	Cough to some degree	Pregnancy
Epilepsy, neuropathic pain	Antiepileptic drug	Topiramate	25–200 mg/d	Weight loss; paresthesias (50%), mnestic deficits (7%)	Pregnancy, kidney stones
Epilepsy, neuropathic pain	Antiepileptic drug	Lamotrigine (only in migraine with aura)	50–300 mg/d	If titrated slowly, well tolerated except skin rashes, rarely Stevens–Johnson syndrome	Idiosyncrasy
Constipation, pediatric migraine	Mitochondrial enhancer	Magnesium	24 mmol/d in adults	Diarrhea	Diarrhea
Anorexia	Ca channel blocker	Flunarizine	10 mg/d	Weight gain, sedation, depression, extrapyramidal side effects	Pregnancy. Parkinson's, history of depression
Comorbid cluster headache, diarrhea, arterial hypertension	Ca channel blocker	Verapamil	80–680 mg/d	Constipation, cardiac	Cardiac conduction problems
Failure of all other therapeutic trials	Serotonin antagonists	Methysergide	1–16 mg/d	Fibrotic disorders with chronic use (break for 1 month after 6 months if treatment)	Fibrotic disorders
Depression, anxiety, neuropathic pain	Antidepressants	Amitriptyline or nortriptyline	10–150 mg/d Start 10mg at bedtime; increase 10mg every 2 weeks; usual dose: 1 mg/kg/d	Dry mouth, weight gain, sedation	Anticholinergic, narrow-angle glaucoma, urinary retention, pregnancy, lactation
Depression, anxiety, neuropathic pain	Antidepressants	Venlafaxine	75–225 mg/d	Nausea	Age under 18 years
None	Mitochondrial enhancer	Vitamin B_2 (riboflavin)	400 mg-0-0	GI side effects in ~3% (diarrhea, flatulence) yellow urine	None
None	Mitochondrial enhancer	Coenzyme Q10	300 mg/d	None	None

Table 10.2 Reciprocal effects of migraine (MIG) and comorbidity (COMORB) therapies and their influence on adjustment of management strategies (+ beneficial effect; = no effect; – deleterious effect).

Therapeutic strategies based on the reciprocal effects of migraine and comorbid disorder therapies			
Effect of migraine therapy on *comorbid* disorder	**Effect** *of comorbid disorder therapy* **on migraine**		
	+	=	–
+	1 THERAPY *may suffice*	MIG THER (add *COMORD THER* if necessary)	MIG THER and Change *COMORB THER*
=	COMORB THER (add MIG THER if necessary)	MIG THER and COMORB THER	Change *COMORB THER*
–	*COMORBID THER* and Change MIG THER	Change MIG THER	Change MIG and *COMORBID THER*

disorder and monotherapy is sufficient to manage both conditions. This might occur in depressed migraineurs in whom both migraine and depression are satisfactorily improved by a tricyclic antidepressant. At the other end of the spectrum (Table 10.2, third line, third column – 'red light'), the antimigraine therapy can worsen the comorbid disorder and vice versa. This could be the case in a depressed migraineur who receives flunarizine, which can worsen depression, or an SSRI (selective serotonin reuptake inhibitor) such as fluoxetine, which can worsen migraine. If this happens, both treatments need to be modified. If the preventive treatment of first choice for migraine has no therapeutic effect for the comorbid disorder (e.g. use of a beta-blocker in a migraineur who also has depression) or if monotherapy is not sufficient (e.g. tricyclic antidepressant is effective for the patient's migraine but not for his depression; Table 10.2, second line, second column – 'orange light'), the patient obviously needs treatment with two distinct medications targeting each disorder.

References
1 Silberstein SD, Goadsby PJ. Migraine: preventive treatment. Cephalalgia 2002;22:491–512.
2 Dodick DW, Silberstein SD. Migraine prevention. Pract Neurol 2007;7:383–93.
3 Silberstein SD, Dodick DW, Freitag F, et al. Pharmacological approaches to managing migraine and associated comorbidities – clinical considerations for monotherapy versus polytherapy. Headache 2007;47:585–99.

Index

Page numbers in *italics* denote figures and tables.

ADHD *See* attention deficit
  hyperactivity disorder
American migraine prevalence and
  prevention (AMPP) study, 114
anxiety disorders
  case report, 2, 129–30
  children, 128
  depression, 6–8
  migraine patients, 3
  'syndromic relationship', 128–9
atherosclerosis risk in communities
  study, 16
attention deficit hyperactivity disorder
  (ADHD), 126
aura without headache, 72
autosomal dominant vascular
  retinopathy, 18

basilar-type migraine, 71–2
benign paroxysmal vertigo, 72

CADSIL, 18, 21
cardio- and cerebrovascular
  disorders
  congenital heart defects, 123
  diagnosis and management
    risk, 35–6
    stroke/MI, 36
  epidemiology
    cardiovascular disease risk, *27–8*
    migraine and cardiovascular risk,
      33–4

triptans and cardiovascular risk,
  31–2
women's and physicians' health
  study, 29–31
Framingham-risk, 19, 34
ischemic stroke, 19
pathophysiology
  endothelial dysfunction (ED), 34
  endothelial progenitor cells
    (EPCs), 34–5
PFO, 123–4
central convergence theory, 86–8
childhood periodic syndromes, 72
children, migraine comorbidities
  ADHD, 126–7
  anxiety disorders, 128–9
  asthma and allergic disorders, 123
  cardiovascular disease, 123–4
  case reports, 129–30
  depression, 127–8
  epilepsy and obesity, 125
  Gilles de la Tourette syndrome, 127
  learning disabilities, 126
  medical and psychiatric, 122
  pathophysiology, 122
  sleep disorders
    management, 126
  stroke, 124
chronic daily headache
  drugs, *102*
  MOH, 100, 106
  obesity, 113–14

Comorbidity in Migraine, First Edition. Edited by J. Schoenen, D. W. Dodick and P. S. Sándor.
© 2011 Blackwell Publishing Ltd. Published 2011 by Blackwell Publishing Ltd.

prevalence, adolescents, 98
TMD symptoms, 117–18
cortical spreading depression (CSD),
     18, 19, 46, 65
confusional migraine, 71–2

depression
    antidepressants, 135
    bipolar subtype, 2–3
    SMILE study, 6–8

electroencephalogram (EEG)
    migraine and epilepsy, diagnosis
        aura, 69–70
        ictus, 70
        postdrome/post-ictal phase, 70
        premonitory phase, 69
        seizure-associated headache, 71
    rhythmic seizure discharge, *60, 61*
epilepsy
    antiepileptic drugs (AEDs), 125
    aura
        definition, 69–70
        description, 69
        visual hallucinations, 70
    case study, Marlie with MA
        EEG, rhythmic seizure discharge,
           59–61
        treatment, 59
    diagnosis and classification
        children, 67
        differential and concomitant,
           EEG, 68–71
        EEG, 71
        ictal progression and symptoms,
           67, *68*
        MA *vs.*, *68*
        primary headaches, 66–7
        seizures and epileptic
           syndromes, 67
        syndromes, 72–3
        variants, 71–2
    epidemiology
        MA and MO, 63
        prevalence, 62–3
    ictus, headache/seizure phase, 70
    occurrence, 62
    pathophysiology
        risk factors, 64–6
        unidirectional causal models, 63
    postdrome/post-ictal phase, 70
    post-ictal, 72

premonitory phase, 69
seizure-associated headache, 71
treatment
    acute and preventive
       modalities, 74
    concomitant diagnoses, 73
    tricyclic antidepressants and
       neuroleptic drug, 73–4

Gastaut syndrome, 73
genetic epidemiology of migraine
     (GEM) study, 33
genetic risk factors, migraine and
     epilepsy
    brain substrate
        epileptogenesis, 64–5
        seizures, 64
    FHM genes
        ATP1A2, 65–6
        CACNA1A, 65
        SCN1A, 66
Gilles de la Tourette syndrome, 127

headache terminators, 102, 104

International Classification of
     Headache Disorders (ICHD-2)
    confusional migraine, 71–2
    migrainous infarction, 17
    migralepsy, 72
International Headache Society (IHS),
     96–7, 114
International League Against Epilepsy
     (ILAE), 62, 67
intranasal contact points
    headache frequency and scores,
       119–20
    mucosal contact headache, 119

learning disabilities (LD)
    causes of, 126
    prevalence, US children, 126
low-dose aspirin therapy, 21–2

MA *See* migraine with aura
medication overuse headache (MOH)
    characteristics, *100*
    description, 96
    diagnosis
        ergot, 100–101
        triptans, 101
    epidemiology

medication overuse headache (*cont'd*)
  analgesics, 97
  drug-induced, 97–8
  population-based studies, 98
  primary headache, 98
  IHS criteria, *97*
  management
    detoxification, 102, 104
    drug withdrawal, 103
    episodic headache, 102
    headache terminators, 104–5
    hospitalization, 103–4
    inpatient headache
      treatment, 104
    preventive treatment, 101
    prophylactic drugs, *102*
    psychiatric illness, 101
    symptoms, 102–3
    topiramate, 101–2
  occurrence, 96–7
  pathophysiology
    chronic daily headache
      (CDH), 99
    5-hydroxytryptamine (5-HT),
      99–100
    mammalian nervous system, 99
    migraineurs, 98–9
    non-migraineurs, 98
    rostral ventromedial medulla
      (RVM), 99
  prevention, 105
  prognosis
    CDH, 106
    withdrawal therapy, 105–6
methylenetetrahydrofolate reductase
    enzyme *(MTHFR C677T)*
  homocysteine, 20, 33
  homozygosity and migraine, 33–4
  replication, 34
migraine-epilepsy syndromes
  benign rolandic epilepsy, 73
  childhood benign partial, occipital
    paroxysms
    Gastaut, 73
    Panayiotopoulos, 72–3
  migraine-triggered seizure, 72
Migraine Intervention with STARFlex©
    Technology (MIST) trial, 20
migraine with aura (MA)
  CVD, 31
  and epilepsy
    comorbidity, 63

  definition, 69–70
  symptoms, *68*
  Framingham risk, 34
  ischemic stroke, 15–17
    mechanism, 27
    women, 19
  and MO, *50*
  MTHFR C677T, 20
  myocardial infarction and
    cardiovascular death, 18–19
  PFO, 123–4
  visual hallucinations, 70
migraine without aura (MO)
  case report, 1–2
  ischemic stroke, 15
  and MA, *50*
  PFO, 45
mitochondrial myopathy,
    encephalopathy, lactacidosis
    and stroke (MELAS), 18
MO *See* migraine without aura
MOH *See* medication overuse
    headache

N-methyl-D-aspartate receptors
    (NMDAR), 99

obesity
  AMPP study, 114–15
  BMI, episodic and chronic
    migraine, 113, *114*
  CDH, 113–14
  children, 125
  clinical intervention, 116
  and migraine population studies, *115*
  weight change, 115–16

pain disorders and migraine
  case presentation
    history, 81
    primary comorbidity, 82
    prophylactic medication, 82
    treatment, 81–2
  comorbidity, 83
  diagnosis and patient handling
    musculoskeletal system, 91–2
    primary and secondary
      headache, 91
    prophylactic drugs, 92
  headaches, comorbidity
    adults, *85*
    children, 84

and chronic musculoskeletal
pain, *85–6*
TTH, 83–4
mechanisms, comorbidity
and blood pressure, *89*
central convergence theory, 87, *88*
factor/disposition, 88–9
hyperexcitability, 87–8
hypertension-related hypalgesia,
89–91
neural mechanism, 87
peripheral triggering theory, 86
pulse pressure level, *90*
systolic blood pressure (SBP), 91
Panayiotopoulos syndrome, 72–3
patent foramen ovale (PFO)
anatomy
description, 42
diagnosis, 43, 44
right-to-left shunt, 42, 44
case report, headache
MRI scan, 41–2
triptan, 41
closure and migraine
MA and MO, 49, *50*
recall bias, 49–50
sham-controlled trial, 50–51
general population
migraine, 45
prevalence, 44, *45*
low-grade evidence linking
migraine, 19–20
and migraine
cardiac disease, 48
characteristics, 51–2
coincidental relationship, 49
cortical spreading depression
(CSD), 46
description, 46
'dose-response' relationship, 47–8
hypercoagulable state, 53–4
MA, 45–6, 48
pulmonary arteriovenous
malformations (AVMs), 48
right-to-left shunting, 46
serotonin, 46–7
stroke, deep white matter (WM)
lesions, 52–3
treatment, 54
in migraineurs
odds ratio (OR), 44–5
prevalence, *45*

migraine with aura, 19
MIST trials, 20
recommendations, migraine
patient, 51
pathophysiology, migraine and stroke
cardiovascular risk factors
with aura, 18–19
ischemic stroke, 19
myocardial infarction, 18
RR, 19
cerebral ischemia, 18
distinct disorders, 18
genetic polymorphisms, 20
ischemic vascular events, 17–18
migrainous infarction, 17
PFO (*see* patent foramen ovale)
postmenopausal hormone
replacement, 18
treatments
ergots use, 20
triptan therapy, 20–21
peripheral triggering theory, 86
PFO *See* patent foramen ovale
probable migraine with visual aura
(PMVA), 124
psychiatric comorbidity
affective disorders
depression, 2
mood, 2–3
symptoms, 3
anxiety disorders
and depression, 3
panic attacks, 3
perfectionism and
obsessionality, 3
case report
acute antimigraine drugs, 2
anxiety, 1–2
hypersomnia, abulia and
anhedonia, 2
medication overuse headache
(MOH), 1
treatment approach, 10
impact
acute antimigraine
medications, 8
anxiety and depression, 8
disability, 6, 8
FRAMIG study, *6–7*
SMILE, *7*
management
antiepileptic drugs, 9

psychiatric comorbidity (*cont'd*)
  behavioral treatments, 9
  depression and anxiety, 8
  drugs, 8–9
  monoamine oxidase inhibitors
    (MAOIs), 9
  preventive therapy, 132
  tricyclic antidepressants, 9
  mechanisms
    anxiety disorders, 5
    factors, 4
    and headache frequency, 5–6
    monoamine systems/
      channelopathies, 6
  substance dependence
    MOH, 4
    nicotine, alcohol and illicit drugs,
      3–4
    painkillers and barbiturates, 4

Raynaud phenomenon, 18
relaxation therapy, 10, 104

sleep disorders, 125–6
stroke and migraine
  brain cells and artery dysfunction, 14
  diagnosis, 21
  epidemiology
    atherosclerosis risk in
      communities study, 16
    diagnoses, 16–17
    hemorrhagic and ischemic
      stroke, 17
    ischemic, risk, 15

migraineurs, aura, 15–16
  stroke prevention in young
    women study, 16
management
  aura features, 22
  low-dose aspirin therapy, 21–2
  traditional risk factors, 21
pathophysiology
  cardiovascular risk factors, 18–19
  cerebral ischemia, 18
  distinct disorders, 18
  genetic polymorphisms, 20
  ischemic vascular events, 17–18
  migrainous infarction, 17
  PFO (*see* patent foramen ovale)
  postmenopausal hormone
    replacement, 18
  treatments, 20–21
probable migraine with visual aura
  (PMVA), 124
stroke prevention in young women
  study, 16

temporomandibular disorders (TMD)
  characterization, 117
  description, 116
  and migraine
    comorbidity, 117
    influence, 117–18
    treatment of, 118–19

unidirectional causal models, 63

withdrawal therapy, *103*, 106